COLD
CURES

COLD CURES

Michael Castleman

FAWCETT COLUMBINE / NEW YORK

A Fawcett Columbine Book
Published by Ballantine Books

Copyright © 1987 by Michael Castleman
Foreword copyright © 1987 by Lisa Johnson, M.D.

All rights reserved under International and Pan-American Copyright Conventions. Published in the United States by Ballantine Books, a division of Random House, Inc., New York, and simultaneously in Canada by Random House of Canada Limited, Toronto.

Library of Congress Catalog Card Number: 86-92118

ISBN: 0-449-90225-0

Text design by Mary A. Wirth

Cover design by Andrew Newman

Manufactured in the United States of America
First Edition: October 1987
10 9 8 7 6 5 4

For Jeffrey Simons Castleman
who must learn to deal with these pesky viruses

Contents

Note

The vast majority of colds may be treated at home without consulting a health professional. However, this book is not in any way intended to substitute for appropriate medical care. Those over seventy, or under ten, or those who are pregnant or nursing or who have heart disease, asthma, emphysema, diabetes, liver disease, serious allergies, a history of stroke, or other chronic health problems should consult a physician before using self-care treatments. Also, consult a physician promptly for any of the symptoms discussed in chapters 17 and 18.

Foreword

If you'd like to save time, money, and a lot of aggravation, I have a suggestion: Learn self-care for the common cold. Ninety-nine times out of a hundred, you can deal with this all-too-common illness without consulting a physician.

Cold self-care also contributes to the public health. Once you understand how colds are transmitted, you can often avoid getting them and giving them to others—at home, at school, and at work. And if everyone learned when the common cold truly required a physician's attention, the nation would take a big step toward better use of its medical resources.

Unfortunately, most people don't know enough about the common cold to care for themselves effectively. They either reach for overpriced remedies they've seen on TV, which may or may not help, or visit physicians seeking antibiotics, which are useless except in the small fraction of cases involving bacterial complications.

The book you hold in your hands puts an end to the confusion. *Cold Cures* represents the state of the art in cold self-care. It covers everything you need to know: what colds are, preventive measures, and the best orthodox medical treatments. It also contains fascinating information about the latest developments in cold research and thorough, clear, and evenhanded discussions of alternative cold treatments. *Cold Cures* is practical, sensible, and reassuring. It's also fun. Once you've read it, you'll know everything your physician knows about the common cold—probably more. Because of *Cold Cures,* I now treat my own colds differently—and more effectively. I'm confident that you will, too.

—Lisa Johnson, M.D.
  Board-Certified Family Practitioner
  Assistant Clinical Professor, Family and Community
  Medicine, University of California, San Francisco

Acknowledgments

For invaluable assistance, I would like to thank my wife, Anne Simons, M.D., assistant clinical professor, family and community medicine, University of California, San Francisco, Calif.; my editors at Ballantine Books, Michelle Russell and Joelle Delbourgo; my agents John Brockman and Katinka Matson, of John Brockman and Associates; my brother and editor-extraordinaire, David Castleman, managing editor, Moon Publications, Chico, Calif.; my colleagues at *Medical Self-Care* magazine: Carole Pisarczyk, Tom Ferguson, M.D., Ted Siff, Lila Purinton, Kerry Tremain, Bobbie Hasselbring, Neshama Franklin, Norma Ashby, Dewey Livingston, Kathryn LeMieux, and Mara Prokop; and all the researchers, practitioners, and consultants who shared their findings, experience, and insights: Robert M. Chanock, M.D., Laboratory of Infectious Diseases, National Institutes of Health, Bethesda, Md.; Robert B. Couch, M.D., professor of Microbiology and Immunology, Baylor College of Medicine, Houston, Tex.; Elliot C. Dick, Ph.D., professor of Preventive Medicine and chief, Respiratory Virus Research Laboratory, University of Wisconsin, Madison; James A. Duke, Ph.D., U.S. Department of Agriculture, Washington, D.C.; George Eby, Austin, Tex.; Joe and Teresa Graedon, co-authors of the *People's Pharmacy* books; Jack M. Gwaltney, Jr., M.D., Frost Professor of Medicine and chief, Division of Epidemiology and Virology, University of Virginia, Charlottesville; Owen Hendley, professor of Pediatrics, University of Virginia, Charlottesville; the staff of the Institute for the Advancement of Health, New York, N.Y.; Dr. Ho Wingtong, Min An Health Center, San Francisco, Calif.; Lisa Johnson, M.D., assistant clinical professor, Family and Community Medicine, University of California, San Francisco, Calif.; Karl Kappus, Ph.D., Centers for Disease Control, Atlanta, Ga.; Anne Linblad, Oriental Healing Arts Institute, Long Beach, Calif.; Hanmin Liu, president, U.S.-China Educational Institute, San Francisco, Calif.; Jean Maguire, health editor, *Redbook* magazine, New York, N.Y.; Jack and Edie Marglon, computer life-savers, San Francisco, Calif.; Rod Moser, Ph.D., professor, Physician Assistant Program, University of California, Davis; Brian Murphy, M.D., Laboratory for Infectious Diseases, National Institutes of Health, Bethesda, Md.; Wendy Murphy, author, *Coping with the Common Cold;* Maryann Napoli, Center for Health Consumers, New York, N.Y.; Planetree Health Resource Center, San Francisco, Calif.; Carolyn Reuben, C.A., Los Angeles, Calif.; Lynda Sadler, Traditional Medicinals, Rohnert Park, Calif.; Eleanor Smith, Berkeley, Calif.; David Sobel, M.D., M.P.H., Kaiser-Permanente, San Jose, Calif., and the staff of the Kaiser Cold Self-Care Program, Vallejo, Calif.; Dana Ullman, M.P.H., co-author (with Stephen Cummings, F.N.P.) of

Everybody's Guide to Homeopathic Medicines; Robert G. Webster, Ph.D., Laboratory of Virology and Immunology, Saint Jude Children's Research Hospital, Memphis, Tenn.; and David R. Zimmerman, author of *The Essential Guide to Nonprescription Drugs.*

COLD
CURES

1,000,000,000 *Colds* *a Year Are* *Nothing to Sneeze At*

Cold Cures is a comprehensive self-care guide to humanity's number-one ailment. The common cold accounts for more illness than *all other diseases combined.* Colds are rarely medically serious, but they cost the nation 30 million lost school and work days a year. Americans spend an estimated $5 billion annually on their colds—$3 billion on cold-related professional consultations and $2 billion on treatment, everything from tissues and vitamin C to over-the-counter drugs and herb teas. Much of that money is wasted. Meanwhile, few people understand that simple preventive measures and self-treatment options really help prevent colds and hasten recovery—some would say cure them.

Cold self-care pays. In a 1983 study in the *Journal of the American Medical Association,* family practitioners at an 875-

family clinic provided half of their patients with some of the information contained in this book—what colds are, the orthodox medical approach to treatment, and guidelines for seeking professional care. Compared with controls who received no self-care information, the test group made 44 percent fewer clinic visits for colds and flu, yet experienced no higher rate of complications. Fewer visits meant significant cost savings for the self-care families and the clinic.

About 5 percent of Americans—some 12 million people—are in some stage of a cold at any given time. In other words, you have a one-in-twenty chance of having a cold right now. But depending on the season, and one's age, medical history, stress level, and contact with young children or their caretakers, risk varies from as high as one in four among infants in day care, to as low as one in one hundred among the healthy elderly (see chapter 4). Whatever your risk, chances are that within the last year you had anywhere from one to six colds. And you probably uttered some variation of that popular lament, "If they can put a man on the moon, why can't they cure the common cold?"

Well, maybe they can. In fact, advocates of several of the cold-care approaches discussed in this book believe they *already have.* You'll have to judge for yourself whether any healing art, orthodox or alternative, has what you consider to be a cure for the common cold, but in the process, I am confident that you'll learn enough about humanity's leading illness to spend a good deal less of your time and money dealing with it.

"Contempt"

Sir William Osler, a noted nineteenth-century physician and medical philosopher, once wrote, "There is just one way to treat the common cold—with contempt." The main reason why colds spread so insidiously and cause so much misery is that people have followed Osler's recommendation. As a nation, we don't take colds seriously enough. We throw billions of dollars at them and argue about vitamin C, but on some level, colds seem to inspire a strange, almost inexplicable national *machismo.* We Americans take perverse pride in denying our colds, unless they become particularly severe. We go to work and increasingly send our children to day care and school despite cold symptoms. To call in sick for "just a cold" somehow suggests weakness of character or moral failing. In many occupations, it's considered bad form, in fact, malingering, to take time off because of a cold.

Commercial cold-formula advertising fuels this cultural attitude. One leading multisymptom remedy promises to "get you through your day." Perhaps, but in the process, you release millions of virus particles and may well infect many other people. The pharmaceutical companies sell more drugs, but where does this denial of colds leave the rest of us? With more colds. Europeans are often amazed that Americans insist on dragging themselves to work, school, or social engagements despite their colds. In many other countries, it's considered rude to co-workers, schoolmates, and friends to expose them to one's virus.

Of course, colds are nowhere near as serious as, say, heart disease, cancer, or stroke, but it's a mistake to dismiss an upper respiratory infection as "just a cold." Childhood colds often progress to ear infections, which may become chronic and cause permanent hearing impairment. Other potential cold complications, particularly pneumonia, may be life-threatening for children, the elderly, and those with other illnesses (see chapter 17). In addition, several possibly life-threatening diseases, particularly influenza A, may initially be mistaken for the common cold. The combination of this "cold counterfeit" and its major complication, pneumonia, ranks as the nation's *fifth leading cause of death,* claiming more than fifty thousand lives annually, and sometimes many more (see chapter 18).

Off Our Knees

Cold Cures is the result of my three years of reporting on the common cold and related illnesses as editor of *Medical Self-Care* magazine (see Appendix). The magazine's mission is to empower the public to stay healthy, take greater responsibility for their health, and assume a more assertive role in their health care when they fall ill. *MSC*'s motto is, It's not enough for doctors to stop playing God. The rest of us must get up off our knees.

Medical Self-Care believes in medical pluralism: No single healing art—neither orthodox nor alternative—has all the answers. At *MSC* we have always recognized that a treatment that works well for one person might not work as well—or even at all—for someone else. The effectiveness of any healing art often depends as much on the individual as on the therapy. As a result, *MSC* tries not to take sides in today's often acrimonious medical controversies, where practitioners of one healing art accuse all others of "quackery," only to be called "charlatans" in return by those they criticize. Although no single healing art has all the answers, most have some good answers to a certain number of common health concerns. *Medical Self-Care* views every healing art—both orthodox and alternative—with skeptical support. Like the magazine, *Cold Cures* believes that healers should "first, do no harm." Beyond that, this book provides options, not prescriptions, and urges readers to keep open minds—to experiment for themselves and come up with the approaches that work best for them.

Of course, when one professes "malice toward none and charity toward all," one runs the risk of alienating *everyone.* Supporters of orthodox Western medicine may be horrified by *Cold Cures'* discussion of vitamin C, as well as herbal, Chinese, and homeopathic cold cures. Similarly, alternative practitioners may feel equally antagonized by the book's discussion of commercial cold formulas and other over-the-counter drugs. So be it. Since its founding in 1976, *Medical Self-Care* has happily endured attacks by aficionados of every healing art for our critical support of every other healing art, and if anything, our commitment to medical pluralism has grown stronger.

Although the various healing arts continue to call each other nasty names, over the last decade, the editors of *Medical Self-Care* have felt encouraged by two key trends reflected in this book. The first is that increasingly health-sophisticated consumers are no longer content to remain passive drones who obey physicians' "orders" without question. Today, health consumers insist on being equal partners in their care. They have also become more aware of the limits of the various healing arts and often prefer to combine them in ways that were unheard of ten years ago.

This transformation of consumer attitudes—and practitioners' deeper appreciation of their own limitations—have fueled the second key trend: the realization that the various healing arts often work better together than separately. A decade ago, most M.D.'s scoffed at chiropractic, acupuncture, meditation, hypnosis, biofeedback, visualization, and nutritional approaches to illness prevention and healing. Today, for many health problems, these approaches are fast becoming the standard of care. Similarly, alternative practitioners who once scoffed at orthodox drugs and surgery have become more open to these approaches for the treatment of many acute illnesses.

My intent is to build on these trends, to empower you to deal more effectively with the common cold by presenting *everything* that may help without doing harm.

1

2,000 Years of Cold Cures

During your last cold, if you took any of the multisymptom cold formulas advertised on television, you may well have used ephedra, the world's oldest cold remedy. The actual drug in commercial cold remedies is ephedra's synthetic equivalent, pseudoephedrine, but it's widely used today for the same reason the ancient Chinese began using it around the time Hippocrates founded Western medicine. Chinese herbalists discovered that a tea brewed with the branches of the shrub they called mahuang was a powerful decongestant that relieved stuffiness due to colds, allergies, and asthma (see chapter 12). Ephedra is native not only to China but also to the American Southwest. During the last century, the pioneers used it extensively, and throughout this country ephedra is still known as Mormon tea (see chapter 11).

Ephedra's effectiveness stands in marked contrast to

many of the other cold remedies our ancestors used. Hippocrates called the common cold *katarrh* from the Greek *katarrhein* for "flowing down," as in mucus from a runny nose. The Greeks believed that colds were caused by excess waste matter in the brain and that nasal secretions eliminated the excess and restored harmony. They were wrong about wastes in the brain, but they were on the right track about the function of nasal mucus (see chapter 3). Unfortunately, in an effort to hasten recovery from colds, most Greek physicians prescribed bleeding. Hippocrates himself advised against bloodletting, but bleeding remained a standard treatment (with or without leeches) for colds and all manner of illnesses well into the nineteenth century.

Pliny the Elder, the Roman naturalist who died in Pompei during the eruption of Mount Vesuvius in A.D. 79, recommended "kissing the hairy muzzle of a mouse."

The tribes of New Guinea covered cold sufferers with large shields painted with symbolic representations of ancestral spirits thought to be capable of warding off the illness. The Chaco Indians of South America performed ceremonial dances in which they threatened cold-causing demons with spears.

And Moses Maimonedes, a twelfth-century rabbi/scholar/physician in Cairo, Egypt, recommended "soup from a fat hen." Chicken soup has been a popular cold remedy ever since, and recent research suggests that it provides some benefit (see chapter 10).

"God Bless You"

Throughout the Middle Ages, the Catholic Church urged cold sufferers to pray for deliverance and condemned many popular folk remedies of the time as witchcraft. It now turns out that prayer and other forms of meditative relaxation may, in fact, help (see chapter 6), but priestly exhortations did not keep superstitious Europeans from believing that upper respiratory infections could lead to demonic possession. Sneezes were considered particularly dangerous because they were thought to expel part of the soul and allow demons to rush in through the mouth. Fortunately, there were two ways to prevent this terrible fate. Sneezers could cover their mouths, which prevented the soul's escape. Or someone nearby could pronounce the demon-defeating benediction "God bless you." Both customs survive to this day. Physicians eventually endorsed covering the mouth for hygienic reasons, but this occurred after the custom had been practiced for centuries.

Priests were also unable to prevent folk healers from prescribing such cold remedies as garlic and onion necklaces, hot foot baths, a variety of medicinal herb teas (see chapter 11), mustard plasters, fish liver oil, throat wraps of salted herring, even sandwiches of cold sufferers' hair placed between bread and fed to dogs.

Another medieval cold cure that still survives in parts of Greece, Mexico, and Southeast Asia is "dry cupping." Lighted candles are placed on the cold sufferer's back and covered with small jars. As the candles consume the oxygen in the jars and go out, they create a partial vacuum which draws the skin underneath up into the jar, producing a warm, stinging sensation. Dry cupping and mustard plasters are "counterirritants." They have no medicinal value, but the irritation they cause temporarily distracts cold sufferers from their discomfort.

During the nineteenth century, most Americans treated their colds with whiskey (see chapter 10), herbs (see chapter 11), and two innovative newcomers to the medical scene—patent medicines and home medical devices. The former, precursors of today's multisymptom cold formulas, included dozens of different pills, salves, plasters, elixirs, and tonics. Some contained potentially helpful herbs, but most relied on copious amounts of alcohol or narcotics (codeine or morphine).

One look at the claims made by these early over-the-counter drugs shows why Congress established the Food and Drug Administration to regulate the drug industry. For example, Tyler's Cherokee Remedy, largely morphine, claimed it could cure colds, coughs, hoarseness, asthma, bronchitis, croup, and whooping cough—even tuberculosis! But these extravagant—and by today's standards, illegal—claims were modest compared with those made by Dr. R. V. Pierce's Golden Medical Discovery. Dr. Pierce asserted that his Discovery provided an "immediate and permanent cure" for every respiratory disease. The patient "finds his whole person entirely renovated and repaired. He feels like a new man—a perfect being." Most of these patent medicines simply stupefied their users while taking credit for the body's own self-healing powers. The best that can be said for them is that they promoted rest.

Among the most popular nineteenth-century home medical devices for the common cold was the nasal douche, a large syringelike affair used to squirt seawater or herbal tonics into the nostrils. Also popular were inhalers, nostril-sized tubes attached to cans or jars filled with aromatic "vapors." Several aromatic remedies for coughs and nasal congestion are still used today (see chapter 11)—minus the often bizarre-looking devices that contained them. One cold-comforting device proved remarkably effective and continues to be widely recommended for cold self-care— the steam-mist vaporizer (see chapter 8).

Today, of course, we view cold remedies such as nasal douches, herring throat wraps, and dry cupping with wry amusement. After all, we're so much more medically sophisticated now. Or are we? In 1966 a leading pharmaceutical company commissioned a survey of Americans' recommendations for preventing and treating the common cold. The suggestions, reportedly offered in all seriousness, included: Drink hot beer. Eat raw peanuts. Avoid wheat and rye. Drink buttermilk with soda water. . . .

C H A P T E R
2

200 Illnesses
Called "Colds"

Most Americans are familiar with the multitalented Benjamin Franklin. He was the statesman who helped draft the Declaration of Independence, the scientist whose kite proved that lightning was electrical, and the author/publisher of *Poor Richard's Almanac* ("Early to bed, early to rise . . ."). However, few know that the Sage of Philadelphia also launched the scientific study of the common cold.

For fifteen hundred years, from the time of the Greek physician Galen (A.D. 130–200) through the 1700s, physicians believed that colds were "phlegmatic" conditions involving inflammation and excess mucus, caused by chilly, damp weather—hence the English term *cold.* Franklin used some homespun epidemiology to challenge the conventional wisdom and arrived at a different—and surprisingly insightful—conclusion.

"Travelling in severe Winters," he wrote, "I have suffered Cold sometimes to an Extremity only short of Freezing, but this did not make me *catch Cold.*" He was equally skeptical of the presumed connection between colds and dampness. An enthusiastic swimmer, he noted: "I have been in the River every Evening for two or three hours. One should suppose that I might imbibe enough damp to *take Cold* if Humidity could give it; but no such effect followed." His skepticism about humidity as a cause of colds was reinforced by his knowledge of the human body. "A Body filled with watery Fluids from Head to Foot cannot be hurt by a little Addition of Moisture."

Once he'd disproved the prevailing view to his own satisfaction, Franklin made a shrewd guess at the true mechanism of contagion. Bear in mind that he lived one hundred years before the discovery of bacteria and the "germ theory," the idea that microorganisms cause illness. Nonetheless, his idea came surprisingly close to the contemporary view. Franklin suggested that colds were caused by "animal substances in the perspired matter from our Bodies [passed] by the frowsy corrupt Air. People often catch colds from one another when shut up together in small close Rooms and Coaches, and when sitting near and conversing so as to breathe each others' Transpiration."

Always practical, Franklin also proposed his own cold preventive, namely, plenty of fresh air, a remedy he championed with typical evangelistic fervor. In the fall of 1776, as colonial leaders prepared to fight for independence, future president John Adams recorded in his diary that he and Franklin shared a room at an inn. The feisty Philadelphian insisted on sleeping with the window wide open. When Adams protested that the chill night air would surely give them colds, Franklin launched into "a harrangue upon Air and Cold and Respiration and Perspiration," an explanation so complex and boring that Adams fell asleep—with the window still open.

After Franklin, naval physicians corroborated the contagious nature of colds by observing that ships' crews were often free of upper respiratory infections for long periods while at sea, but inevitably developed them shortly after docking.

Then, during the mid-1800s, Louis Pasteur's pioneering work with bacteria popularized the germ theory of illness, and scientists began to blame colds on these microscopic one-celled organisms. Disease-causing bacteria were sometimes found in the respiratory tracts of those with colds, but in 1914, V. W. Kruse, a German researcher, showed that cold sufferers' nasal secretions, carefully filtered to remove all bacteria, could still cause colds when introduced into healthy noses. As a result, the common cold joined a growing number of illnesses—smallpox and influenza, among others—whose transmission did not fit Pasteur's bacterial model. For a while, these diseases were thought to be caused by toxins produced by bacteria, and the word *virus* was coined from the Latin for "poison." The toxin theory proved correct in the case of diphtheria, but as chemical-analysis techniques improved, the other viral illnesses yielded no toxins, and the term *virus* slowly began to be applied to a new class of presumably submicroscopic pathogens.

Despite Kruse's early evidence that a virus caused the common cold, for twenty-four years almost no one in medicine believed him. He was German, and his research at the start of World War I, though translated, was dismissed by most American scientists as the work of "the enemy." In addition, despite frequent headlines announcing medical "breakthroughs," medicine tends to be quite conservative. Many important discoveries take years to become accepted—a fact partisans of vitamin C never tire of pointing out (see chapter 9). Finally, in 1938, A. R. Dochez at Columbia University repeated Kruse's work. His article in the *Journal of the American Medical Association* established the common cold as a viral illness once and for all.

During the 1940s, J. H. Dingle at Case-Western Reserve University in Cleveland showed that the family plays a key role in the spread of colds and that young children, the most susceptible group, are "the primary viral reservoir."

But virology remained a frustrating, hit-and-miss pursuit until 1949, when Boston researcher John Enders developed a reliable technique for growing viruses in the laboratory. Enders won a Nobel Prize, and his work spurred the development, a few years later, of the Salk polio vaccine. It also enabled cold researchers for the first time to attempt to develop a vaccine against what they assumed was a single cold virus.

The eagerly sought cold virus was isolated in 1954 at Tulane University and confirmed shortly after at the Common Cold Research Unit of Harvard Hospital in Salisbury, England, a unique facility still in operation today where healthy volunteers spend ten-day, all-expense-paid "holidays" in exchange for subjecting themselves to experimental colds. The U.S. and British viruses were similar, but oddly, not identical. Then another cold virus was isolated, and another, and scientists soon realized that the common cold was not a single disease caused by a solitary organism, but many different illnesses with remarkably similar symptoms caused by a bewildering variety of viruses.

As the catalogue of cold viruses grew, hopes for a vaccine faded. Vaccines are quite specific. They only work against single organisms (though some may confer partial immunity to others that are closely related). By the early 1960s, dozens of cold viruses had been identified. Today the number is about two hundred and still climbing. Barring a major advance in vaccine technology, it seems extremely unlikely that there will ever be a shot to prevent humanity's leading illness.

Perfect Parasites

Viruses are among the most puzzling life-forms. They are so tiny that if a human red blood cell—itself less than a thousandth of an inch in diameter—were the size of a typical home, a cold virus would be about the size of a window. In many ways, viruses are not even alive. They have no cells, no organs, no brain, nothing except fragments of genetic material (DNA or RNA) inside a rudimentary protein coat. Viruses do not digest food, respire oxygen, grow, eliminate wastes, repair themselves, or interact with their environment like other organisms. Their sole lifelike attribute is the ability to reproduce—an activity they pursue with a vengeance.

Viruses are parasites. They invade specific target cells of their specific hosts—in the case of colds, the epithelial cells that line the human nose and throat (nasopharynx)—then seize control and force these cells to reproduce thousands of new virus particles, a process that kills the host cells.

The major task of life is to reproduce life, but within limits. An organism must reproduce in sufficient quantity to allow the reproductive process to continue, but it must not reproduce so many individuals that their number exhausts the food supply—or, in the case of parasites, the host supply—which would threaten its own species survival.

Parasites may be considered along a continuum from primitive to sophisticated. Primitive parasites reproduce with such virulence that they threaten their own survival by threatening their hosts. They cause symptoms quickly (brief incubation), debilitate the host immediately (limiting transmission), kill a large proportion of hosts quickly (limiting production of new parasites), and have only one host (no fallback if the primary host becomes depopulated). No truly primitive parasite could survive for long.

Advanced parasites are more cunning. They have extended incubation periods, cause only relatively minor symptoms, rarely limit their transmission by overwhelming the host, rarely kill, and have more than one host just in case something else kills off the primary host. By these measures, cold viruses are among the world's most advanced parasites. They offer us a Faustian bargain: generally minor illness with no threat to our species' survival in exchange for maddeningly frequent illness and no threat to their survival. No wonder these sneaky little devils cause more illness than all other germs combined. Cold viruses may rank among the planet's simplest life-forms, but they literally have us by the throat.

"Different Animals"

Seven major viral families cause upper respiratory infections. One causes influenza (see chapter 18), and six cause colds. Some years ago, one cold formula attempted to distinguish itself from the competition by claiming particular effectiveness against summer colds. Its slogan: "A summer cold is a different animal." Viruses are not "animals," but the slogan contains a germ, as it were, of truth. Each cold virus causes a "different" cold, even though the symptoms are usually indistinguishable.

The various viral families also cause different percentages of upper respiratory infections (URIs) and tend to be most active at different times of the year. Studies over the last thirty years suggest the following estimates:

. . .

VIRAL GROUP	PERCENTAGE OF URIs	SEASONALITY
Rhinoviruses	30–50	Spring, summer, fall
Parainfluenza	15–25	Fall, winter, spring
Influenza A and B	10–20*	Late fall, winter, early spring
Coronaviruses	10–20	Winter, spring
Respiratory Syncytial Virus	10	Fall, winter, spring
Enteroviruses	5–10	Spring, summer, fall
Adenoviruses	3–7	Winter
Others	up to 25	Year-round

*More during periodic worldwide epidemics (pandemics)

For convenience of discussion, this book treats "the common cold" as a single illness. But each viral group is unique and, technically speaking, causes different colds:

RHINOVIRUSES. Rhinoviruses cause up to half of all colds. The name comes from the Greek for "nose," the primary site of infection. Scientists have identified one hundred distinct rhinoviruses, many of which have several variants, for a total of more than a hundred and fifteen.

The incubation period lasts from one to four days, usually two. Although symptoms typically appear within forty-eight hours, rhinovirus cold sufferers begin to release ("shed") virus particles within about seven hours, and each infected nasopharyngeal cell produces as many as one thousand virus particles within fifteen hours. In other words, you can catch a rhinovirus cold for *a day and a half before* the person who gives it to you "catches" it. Viral shedding typically peaks by day three or four as the sore throat subsides and the nose becomes congested. However, significant shedding can continue for up to a week after all symptoms have disappeared, and in young children, shedding may continue for up to three weeks. For organisms without brains, these viruses are incredibly sly.

Of course, the body is not without defenses. Spouses transmit rhinovirus colds to each other only about one-third to one-half the time, prompting prominent cold researcher Elliot C. Dick, chief of the Respiratory Virus Research Laboratory at the University of Wisconsin in Madison, to comment that "rhinovirus infections are surprisingly difficult to transmit." That's the good news. The bad news is that although many of the rhinovirus-exposed do not develop full-blown colds but "subclinical infections," (semi-colds with mild symptoms or no symptoms at all), they may still shed enough virus to infect others.

Rhinoviruses cause colds year-round, but they are most active from April through October. In other words, the viral group that causes the most colds is least active from November through March, the height of the annual cold and flu season.

Once infected with any germ, the sufferer's immune system develops antibodies that protect the person from reinfection, ideally for life. Unfortunately, antibodies against cold viruses do not last long. Immunity to rhinoviruses lasts from two to four years, then declines to the point where reinfection becomes possible again. However, even those with lots of antibodies may suffer several colds in rapid succession because many different types of rhinovirus—and other cold viruses—are typically prevalent at any given time. Serial infection is most common among infants and young children, many of whom seem to have colds continually.

Rhinovirus colds usually last for a few days to two weeks, and average about a week. Rhinoviruses do not cause complications as frequently as several other upper respiratory viruses; nonetheless, complications are possible (see chapter 17).

PARAINFLUENZA VIRUSES. This family of four viruses causes 15 to 25 percent of colds. Symptoms are usually mild in adults, but in infants, 75 percent of whom suffer parainfluenza infection by age two, parainfluenza viruses are second only to respiratory syncytial (sin-SISH-al) virus as a cause of cold complications.

Parainfluenza viruses are most active in the fall, winter, and spring. For reasons unknown, since 1980 this virus's peak activity period has shifted from the autumn to the spring.

One type of parainfluenza virus has an "attack rate" of nearly 100 percent, meaning that just about all exposed, antibody-free infants become ill. The other three cause illness in 40 to 70 percent of exposed infants, with progressively lower attack rates as people grow older (except among those who care for infants). Antibody protection is weak. About one-third of infants with parainfluenza antibodies get sick when reexposed. Fortunately, the complication rate decreases with subsequent infections. Reinfection decreases sharply after age two.

Parainfluenza colds incubate longer than rhinovirus colds—two to four days in children, three to six days in adults. Adult shedding usually stops after eight to ten days, but children may shed virus for up to four weeks. Given the extended duration of shedding and the relatively high risk of immediate reinfection, outbreaks of parainfluenza colds can be persistent—and potentially serious—in day-care centers and hospital pediatric units.

CORONAVIRUSES. This family of thirteen viruses, named for its distinctive crowned appearance under the electron microscope, causes a variety of diseases in other mammals, but human coronavirus (HCV) simply causes colds, 10 to 20 percent of upper respiratory infections.

HCV is active in winter and spring, and significant outbreaks typically occur at two-year intervals. Overall, about

15 percent of the population develops a coronavirus cold each year. But during peak months, HCV infection may reach epidemic proportions, accounting for 25 to 30 percent of adult colds.

HCV colds incubate slightly longer than rhinovirus colds (two to five days), but have a similar average duration (seven days). Like rhinovirus colds, however, they may linger for as long as two weeks. Symptoms are similar to rhinovirus colds, but HCV colds are more likely to cause fever and less likely to cause cough.

Unlike most other upper respiratory viruses, children are no more susceptible than adults. In fact, the group at highest risk is young adult military recruits, who apparently become susceptible because of the crowding, stress, and chronic fatigue of basic training.

HCV colds rarely cause complications, except in asthmatic children and military recruits, who may develop bronchitis or pneumonia.

RESPIRATORY SYNCYTIAL VIRUS. RSV accounts for about 10 percent of colds and generally produces only mild symptoms. However, in infants, it's the leading cause of cold complications, including potentially life-threatening pneumonia.

Virtually 100 percent of children suffer RSV infection by age three. Fortunately, the vast majority recover uneventfully from the nasal congestion and runny nose it causes. But up to 20 percent develop complications, and a few suffer pneumonia. About two infants in a thousand must be hospitalized. Deaths from RSV pneumonia are rare but possible. Some research suggests that breast-feeding decreases the risk of RSV complications. Other studies show that parental cigarette smoking increases it.

RSV strikes like clockwork each autumn around Thanksgiving and remains active until April. Most outbreaks peak from December to March.

RSV causes mild colds in adults. The incubation period is about five days, and the illness typically lasts less than a week, though possibly longer in those who care for infants.

Robert M. Chanock, M.D., a leading RSV authority at the National Institute of Allergy and Infectious Diseases in Bethesda, Maryland, calls this virus "a great escape artist," because it has an uncanny ability to elude the immune system's defenses. RSV infection sparks antibody production, but for reasons unknown, immunity disappears within a year, and lifelong reinfection is commonplace. Reinfection rates as high as 74 percent have been recorded in day-care centers.

Because RSV is a single virus, during the 1960s Chanock attempted to develop a vaccine. But in a bizzare twist of fate, when the vaccine was tested, recipients not only remained susceptible to RSV infection, they also experienced unexpectedly severe symptoms, and the vaccine was abandoned. Today, the new antiviral drug, ribavirin (Virazole), has been shown effective against RSV pneumonia.

ENTEROVIRUSES. This group of more than 125 viruses is related to the rhinoviruses and includes the causes of polio and some viral meningitis. Two subgroups cause colds: echoviruses and Coxsackieviruses (named for Coxsackie, New York, where they were first isolated).

Echoviruses and Coxsackieviruses cause 5 to 10 percent of colds. They are active from April through December, with peak activity in the summer and fall. They have the longest incubation period of any upper respiratory virus, typically seven to fourteen days.

Although these colds can strike at any age, like most cold viruses, they cluster among children. About 25 percent of enterovirus colds occur in infants, another 25 percent in children from two to ten. Military recruits also develop a disproportionate share of these infections.

Enteroviruses cause typical cold systems and possibly diarrhea. Complications are rare but possible.

ADENOVIRUSES. Among the more than forty adenoviruses, several cause gastroenteritis ("stomach flu"), and three types account for about 5 percent of colds. Adenoviruses are most active in fall and winter. Unlike most other colds, they shed for only about four days.

Children are only slightly more susceptible than adults. The group at greatest risk is military recruits. For unknown reasons, during the 1950s and 1960s this virus caused virulent epidemics of a flulike illness at several military installations used for basic training. The illness, acute respiratory disease (ARD), struck in winter and at some bases infected 80 percent of recruits, up to half of whom developed pneumonia. Several died. Researchers discovered that ARD was caused by just two strains of adenovirus and developed a vaccine approved in 1971. ARD has not disappeared, but incidence has decreased by more than 50 percent. The vaccine, however, is licensed for use only by the Armed Forces.

OTHER VIRUSES. Scientists estimate that the viruses responsible for up to 25 percent of all colds have not yet been discovered. In recent years, increased attention has been focused on Epstein-Barr virus, a cause of mononucleosis, which also causes a recurring, poorly understood, flulike illness.

As we conclude our tour of "The Wide World of Cold Viruses," bear in mind that throughout the year, many different cold viruses are active at once. Researchers studying a Chicago nursery school discovered fourteen different rhinoviruses during a nine-month period. And an eight-month study of a University of Wisconsin housing development revealed seven different rhinoviruses, two parainfluenza viruses, adenovirus, echovirus, influenza B virus, respiratory syncytial virus, and several unidentified viruses. As one virologist remarked, "God created humanity to provide a good home for cold viruses."

Cold War: The Body as Battleground

With hordes of crafty cold viruses continually poised to make us feel miserable, it's a wonder that only about one person in twenty has a cold at any given time. But after millennia of constant combat with these tiny adversaries, the immune system has evolved astonishingly complex and ingenious defenses against our leading ailment.

The body's first line of defense is the nose itself. Cold viruses reproduce best in dry air (relative humidity below 50 percent) at temperatures slightly below normal body temperature (85° to 95°F). To inhibit viral replication, the nose has a rich blood supply near its inner surface, which moistens incoming air to a relative humidity of about 75 percent and warms it to near body temperature (98.6°). The inner nose also has flaplike "turbinates," which increase its surface area and assist in this warming, moistening process.

As a result, the microenvironment inside the healthy nose and throat is not particularly hospitable to cold viruses.

The nasopharynx is also lined with cells that secrete sticky mucus and have tiny projecting hairs called *cilia*. Like flypaper, the mucus traps inhaled dust, pollen, and microorganisms, preventing them from coming into contact with the cells underneath. The cilia move the mucus and trapped particles down the throat—at a speed of about one inch every five minutes—into the stomach, where powerful digestive acids destroy most germs.

In addition, the cells that line the respiratory tract also secrete a substance called immunoglobulin A (IgA). IgA is one of several immune-system proteins (IgG, IgM, IgE) collectively known as antibodies, which prevent viruses and bacteria from causing infection. Antibodies work at the molecular level. Invading microorganisms have particular surface characteristics that allow them to fit in lock-and-key fashion into molecule-sized receptor sites on the surfaces of their specific target cells. Immunoglobulins, composed of four chains of molecules, wrap around the invaders and, in effect, change their shape so that their surface "keys" no longer fit their target cells' "locks."

Infection

But during a cold, virus particles manage to penetrate the mucous layer, and in those who lack the specific virus IgA, and attach themselves to nasopharyngeal cells. Then molecules in the viruses' protein coats punch holes in the target cell membranes, allowing viral genetic material (DNA or RNA) to enter the cells. Within a short time, the virus seizes control, forcing the production of thousands of new virus particles, which the cold sufferer begins to shed up to several days before any symptoms appear.

On the other side of the battle lines, as nose and throat cells become infected, they release chemicals that marshal the immune system to fight the viral invasion. The immune system is incredibly complex, and scientists still do not fully understand it. However, we know that infection triggers many immune responses simultaneously. The myriad components of the immune system use an amazing amount of teamwork to fight the infection, in much the same way that neighbors, police, various fire departments, the news media, the insurance industry, and government and social service agencies work together to deal with a tornado.

Within an hour of viral infection, the injured cells release chemicals called *prostaglandins,* which trigger inflammation and attract infection-fighting white blood cells called *neutrophils.* Neutrophils, which account for about two-thirds of the body's white blood cells, attempt to engulf the invaders and digest them without attacking the infected cells.

Neutrophil activity stimulates further inflammation. The infected area turns red and swells, and the tiny blood vessels (capillaries) around the infection site stretch (dilate). As the capillaries dilate, their walls come to resemble stretched socks; spaces open up among the "threads" that hold them together. These spaces allow blood fluid (plasma), additional neutrophils, and other specialized white blood cells to flood the area. Plasma, a key factor in the swelling associated with inflammation, also raises the temperature of the infected area, which inhibits viral replication.

Another substance released shortly after infection is *histamine,* which increases nasal mucus secretion in an effort to trap more virus particles before they can attach to target cells. Histamine also increases the capillaries' permeability, which encourages the flow of plasma and white blood cells into the area.

If the neutrophils and increased temperature do not turn the tide against the viral invader, inflammation continues, and within four to five hours, two kinds of specialized white blood cells, *monocytes* and *lymphocytes,* pass through the capillary walls and enter the fray. Monocytes account for about

5 to 10 percent of white blood cells. When they encounter inflammation and other chemical signals of infection, they transform themselves into *macrophages* (literally, "big eaters"), which assist the neutrophils in devouring cold-virus particles. Each macrophage can digest as many as one hundred virus particles. The macrophages also release *interleukin-1,* which signals the brain to raise body temperature and activates the next level of immune response, the lymphocytes.

The Big Guns

Lymphocytes, which account for 20 to 25 percent of white blood cells, are the heavy artillery of the immune system. Ordinarily, most reside quietly in the lymph glands scattered around the body, but when inflammation and other chemical signals summon them to an infection site, they become warrior cells that, in the vast majority of cases, ultimately vanquish the cold virus.

There are two types of lymphocytes: B-cells and T-cells. B-cells, named for the bone marrow where they mature, account for about 3 to 5 percent of white blood cells and produce immunoglobulins, the antibodies that plug the cold-virus receptor sites and prevent them from attaching to nasopharyngeal cells. Some become special "memory cells," which recognize the virus if it invades again and immediately plug the viral receptor sites, thus preventing reinfection.

T-cells, which account for 15 to 20 percent of white blood cells, are produced in the bone marrow, but mature in the thymus, a small gland under the breastbone. When summoned to an infection site, some turn into "killer cells," which attack and destroy virus-infected cells (and some tumor cells). Others become "helper/inducer" cells, which stimulate the B-cells to produce more antibodies. Still others become "suppressor" cells, which shut off antibody production and killer-cell activity after the virus has been defeated.

T-cells also release several substances that help the body fight infection: macrophage activation factor, macrophage migration inhibition factor, interleukin-1 and -2, and interferons. *Macrophage activation factor* stimulates the big-eater cells to devour more virus particles faster. *Macrophage migration inhibition factor* holds the macrophages in the infected area longer than they would stay by themselves. *Interleukin-1* signals the brain to raise body temperature, which impairs viral replication. Elevated body temperature also spurs the T-cells and B-cells to greater virus-fighting activity. *Interleukin-2* further stimulates the B-cells to produce more antibodies. (Genetically engineered interleukin-2 also shows promise as a cancer treatment.)

Interferon (another promising cancer medication) is popularly known as "the body's own antiviral drug." In fact, it is not a single chemical, but at least twenty similar substances which activate the killer cells, and stimulate healthy cells in the infected area to produce "antiviral protein." Cells exposed to the interferons may become infected, but for reasons not yet known, antiviral protein prevents viral replication and cell death.

The final component of the immune arsenal is known as *the complement system,* a noncellular collection of at least twenty proteins, which circulate in blood plasma. Among their many functions, complement proteins coat virus particles, making them easier for macrophages to recognize and digest, and help the killer cells identify infected cells, which must be destroyed.

Symptoms as Defenses

Up to several days before the cold sufferer develops any symptoms, the immune system is locked in mortal combat against the invading viral hordes. Cold viruses may be barely alive, but their ultimate defeat requires the coordinated efforts of an enormous defensive armada: neutrophils, macrophages, B-cells, T-cells, killer cells, immunoglobulins, histamine, postaglandins, interleukin-1 and -2, interferons, the complement system, and many other factors.

Within one to seven days after virus particles first penetrate upper respiratory mucus, the inflammation process progresses to the point where swelling in the nose and throat stimulates nerves in the area to signal the brain that the cold sufferer has a sore throat and perhaps itchy eyes, a headache, or a vague awareness of "a cold coming on."

At the same time, the interleukin-1 released by the macrophages signals the brain to raise body temperature, which inhibits viral replication and stimulates T- and B-cell activity. But body temperature cannot rise as quickly as the brain would like. As a result, the body's complex temperature-sensing mechanism detects a difference between the higher temperature the brain has ordered and actual body temperature, which remains temporarily lower. The brain decides that the body is "too cool" and reacts by stimulating "chills," which typically precede fever.

In addition to triggering chills, interleukin-1 also causes some breakdown of muscle proteins, which the cold or flu sufferer experiences as "muscle aches."

As the Battle of the Nasopharynx rages, some plasma seeps into the mucus-producing tissue that lines the nose and throat, causing it to swell. The cold sufferer experiences this as nasal congestion. Meanwhile, histamine released by the inflammation process stimulates the mucus-secreting cells to increase their production, a process further stimulated by the release of the interferons. However, nasal congestion prevents some of this excess mucus from taking its usual drainage path down the throat and into the stomach. Some plasma-soaked, watery mucus drains out the nose, hence runny nose. Excess mucus and other cold-related irritation in the respiratory tract also trigger sneezing and coughing.

Within a few days after infection, the immune system turns the tide against the cold virus, and usually within a week to ten days, the invader has been destroyed. The inflammation subsides. Mucus production and drainage gradually return to normal. Cold symptoms clear up. And the body's defensive forces return to their various bases in the lymph glands and bloodstream. Although the cold sufferer has felt lethargic and congested for a week, he or she has gained memory-cell antibodies, which prevent reinfection by that particular virus for up to several years. The virus has been destroyed, but the cold sufferer has released millions of new virus particles, which may infect others.

Cold symptoms are certainly annoying, but as we've seen, they are not produced by the virus itself. They result from the immune system's many responses to it. "Cold sufferers feel fine while being infected," Wendy Murphy writes in *Coping with the Common Cold*. "They discover that they have 'just' caught their colds as the body begins to cure them, and feel miserable mainly because the body is making them well."

Susceptibility: Who Catches Colds— and Why

Cold prevention is discussed in chapter 6, but even without taking any precautions, susceptibility varies tremendously. It's based on many factors, several discovered only recently—and some quite surprising.

Chilling and Dampness

Mothers the world over tell their children, "Bundle up or you'll catch your death." They also insist on galoshes and other rain gear because "everyone knows" that damp cold leads to colds. The chill/damp theory is one of the most enduring beliefs about our number-one illness—and the most thoroughly debunked.

Recall that Benjamin Franklin was the first scientist to be left cold by the cold theory of colds. Nobody listened to him. Years later, physicians repeatedly observed that polar explorers developed surprisingly few colds while exposed for months at a time to temperatures as low as −100°F. Again, nobody listened. In the 1930s, epidemiologist Wade Hampton Frost, of Johns Hopkins, correlated infirmary visits for colds with Baltimore temperature and weather patterns and found no association. Nobody believed him, either.

When Britain's Common Cold Research Unit was established in 1946, one of the first experiments devised by director Sir Christopher H. Andrewes was a test of the chill/damp theory. Here's how he described it in 1951 in *Scientific American:*

> To test the practically universal idea that chilling induces colds, we organized three groups of six volunteers. One received a dose of virus. One was given no virus, but its members were severely chilled. After a hot bath, they were made to stand in a drafty passage in wet bathing suits for half an hour, which left them quite cold and miserable. They were also made to wear wet socks the rest of the morning. The third group received the virus plus the chilling treatment. We performed this experiment three times. In not one instance did chilling alone produce a cold. And in two out of three tests, chilling plus virus produced *fewer* colds than virus alone.

Still, the world turned a deaf ear. So in 1958, University of Illinois researchers H. F. Dowling and G. G. Jackson repeated Andrewes's experiment. They had subjects stand either naked in a 60°F room for four hours or clothed in 10°F for two hours. Once chilled, the two groups were inoculated with cold virus. They developed the same number of colds with the same symptom severity as unchilled, virus-inoculated subjects. But the mothers of the world *still* did not listen. So much for science.

There have been a few other tests of the chill/damp

theory these past thirty years. None have shown any relationship to upper respiratory infection. But even the most rigorous research is apparently powerless against "the practically universal idea" that chilling and dampness are a one-way ticket to the common cold. Cold researchers say they don't worry about getting chilled. But privately, one sheepishly conceded that his wife insists that their children bundle up.

Age

Susceptibility to colds definitely decreases with age. Infants typically suffer up to nine colds during their first year. By age three, the number usually drops below six. Teens usually suffer three or four colds annually, after which the number continues to fall until late in life, when the healthy elderly average just one or two a year.

Children have the poorest personal hygiene. To the extent that self-discipline can prevent the spread of colds (see chapter 6), they have the least self-control. Children also have the least immunity to cold viruses. One of the major tasks of childhood is to "exercise" the developing immune system through frequent exposure to colds and other diseases.

There are, however, two exceptions to the rule that susceptibility decreases with age. Parents experience a sharp jump in colds while their children are young, no matter what their own age at the time. And those who spend considerable time with children—elementary teachers, day-care staff, and so on—catch more colds because they are exposed to so many children's cold viruses.

Crowding is also a factor in childhood colds, especially now that so many infants and toddlers are in day care. Crowding facilitates direct contact. Crowding is also a factor in the high incidence of upper respiratory infections among military recruits.

Increasing age often brings less severe colds. During middle age, the inflammation response subsides somewhat, and histamine production declines (which is why many allergy sufferers notice less severe hay fever as they grow older).

Sex

For reasons unknown, boys suffer more colds than girls until age three, after which girls become somewhat more susceptible. Women's greater lifelong susceptibility probably has to do with their role as children's caretakers. In addition, Dowling and Jackson, whose work on chilling was mentioned earlier, also found that reproductive-age women tend to be particularly susceptible to colds around the time of ovulation each month, presumably because of hormonal changes associated with the menstrual cycle.

Income

Colds tend to decrease as income increases. Low-income people are more likely to have more children and live in more crowded circumstances. Low income is also associated with increased stress levels (see below) and with poor diet, which may impair the immune system.

Smoking

The research here is contradictory. Some studies show that cigarettes increase susceptibility to colds; others do not. But the studies all agree that smokers suffer more severe cold symptoms, especially coughing. Smoking irritates the entire respiratory tract and paralyzes the cilia that clear it of mucus. Several studies also show that children of parents who smoke are more susceptible to all respiratory illnesses.

Relative Humidity

Workers in air-conditioned offices often complain of increased susceptibility to colds and sore throats and usually make the mistake of blaming the problem on chilling. The real culprit appears to be the low relative humidity of refrigerated air. Recall that cold viruses are most effective in dry air and that one function of the nose is to moisten incoming breaths. Low relative humidity dries nasal mucus, opening cracks that allow cold viruses to infect exposed cells. In a Canadian study, schools that had relative humidities of 50 percent experienced half as many cold-related absences as those with relative humidities of only 25 percent. And a British researcher writes that low relative humidity "impairs the immune responsiveness of the nasal mucosa, reduces output of IgA, and may increase susceptibility to upper respiratory tract infections."

Other Illnesses

Those whose immune systems are preoccupied with other illnesses show increased susceptibility to upper respiratory infections (and to lower respiratory complications). The same is true for those whose immune systems have been disabled by immunosuppressive drugs, for example, organ transplant recipients. On the other hand, allergies such as hay fever, which cause coldlike nasal symptoms, do not increase susceptibility to colds.

Social Support

The song says, "People who need people are the luckiest people in the world." Recently, scientists have discovered that they are also the healthiest. The importance of "social support systems"—the friends, spouses, relatives, and organizations we sometimes take for granted—was first demonstrated in a 1974 study of heart disease by epidemiologists Lisa Berkman and Leonard Syme of the University of California at Berkeley. They unearthed a detailed health and life-style survey completed nine years earlier by seven thousand residents of one California county and analyzed the responses for diet, obesity, smoking, blood pressure, and cholesterol, the risk factors long considered predictive of heart attacks. On a hunch, they also checked "social connectedness," the amount of time the respondents said they spent with other people. Then the researchers checked the county's death registry to see which respondents had died during the intervening nine years. The results were striking. Independent of all other variables, loners had significantly more fatal heart attacks than their more sociable counterparts. And those with the fewest interpersonal connections were *three times* more likely to die of all causes.

Scientists are still not certain why social isolation is so deadly, but many subsequent studies have shown that it correlates strongly with depression and feelings of hopelessness and helplessness, which, among other effects, decrease IgA levels, and generally impair immune responsiveness.

Since the work of Berkman and Syme, social isolation has been shown to be a risk factor not only for fatal diseases, but also for many nonfatal illnesses—including the common cold. A 1980 study by Richard Totman at the Common Cold Research Unit in England subjected fifty-two volunteers to a comprehensive battery of personality, life-style, and stress tests, then inoculated them with a rhinovirus. When the questionnaires were analyzed for social support, "introverts developed significantly more colds with worse symptoms than extroverts."

At first this might seem odd. Since colds are spread by interpersonal contact (see chapter 5), one might assume that isolation would be protective. *Physical* isolation *is* protective; sailors and Arctic explorers develop few colds. But *emotional* isolation depresses the immune system and significantly increases susceptibility.

Stress

Emotional isolation may not feel anything like getting married, sustaining a serious injury, or commuting in rush-hour traffic, but psychologists consider all four of the above quite stressful. Ever since the 1956 publication of Hans Selye's groundbreaking book, *The Stress of Life,* many health authorities have come to believe that "stress"—everyday anxieties and pressures, and all significant life changes, whether good or bad—is as important to health as "germs" are. A tremendous body of research shows that emotional stress increases the risk of many serious illnesses. Several studies show that the same is true for colds. In the study mentioned earlier, Totman found "a highly significant positive association" between stress and cold susceptibility. Subjects under stress caught more colds and worse colds, "clear evidence of a psychosomatic component in upper respiratory infections."

How Colds Spread:
The Controversy Continues

Pasteur's germ theory of illness gave scientists their first real insight into disease transmission. Like movie detectives in hot pursuit ordering cabbies to "Follow that car," medical researchers threw themselves into following bacteria—and later, viruses—into and out of the body. For upper respiratory infections, the logical germ carriers were the aerosol droplets coughed and sneezed by cold sufferers—what Benjamin Franklin had called "breathing each others' Transpiration."

By Pasteur's time, the medieval custom of covering the mouth while sneezing to keep the soul in and demons out had faded. But with the advent of the germ theory, it suddenly made scientific sense. The real demons were germs, and physicians and arbiters of etiquette quickly joined forces to promote mouth covering during coughs and sneezes in the name of public health. But the repopularization of this custom did not occur overnight. As late as World War II, the British Ministry of Health deemed it necessary to produce a poster headlined, "Coughs and Sneezes Spread Diseases. Trap Germs in Your Handkerchief to Keep the Nation Fighting Fit." It turns out that cloth handkerchiefs are among the *worst* places to trap cold viruses, but scientists did not make this discovery until the 1970s (see chapter 6).

Aerosols Forever?

During the 1930s and 1940s, researchers bolstered the "aerosol transmission theory" by showing that sneeze droplets explode from the mouth at speeds of up to 150 feet per second, can remain aloft for up to several hours, and may travel great distances. The aerosol view gained additional support in the 1950s when studies at Britain's Common Cold Research Unit showed that healthy volunteers could catch rhinovirus colds when they were separated from cold sufferers by a screen.

British cold researchers also investigated the possibility that the hands might pick up enough rhinovirus by "direct contact" during nose blowing to transmit it. Sir Christopher Andrewes describes this early experiment:

> We fixed up a volunteer with an artificial running nose by attaching a small container of liquid to his nose, and letting the liquid drip out at about the rate of secretion a cold might produce. In this liquid was a flourescent dye visible in even tiny traces under ultraviolet light. The subject spent four hours in a room with three others, blowing his nose but otherwise conducting himself in a normal manner. Afterwards, under the ultraviolet lamps, the dye's distribution was quite amazing. Not only was the volunteer's handker-

chief soaked with it, but there were dots of dye all over his face, hands, and clothes—even on the food he was about to eat.

Subsequently, however, British volunteers caught no colds after handling toys used by cold-infected children, and scientists at the Common Cold Research Unit lost interest in direct-contact transmission. The aerosol theory seemed unassailable.

By 1970, however, the aerosol theory had lost its luster. It turned out that rhinovirus cold sufferers' cough and sneeze droplets contain only tiny amounts of live virus. Most of the aerosol spray comes not from the virus-rich nose, but from saliva, which remains relatively virus-free during colds.

Scientists divide cough and sneeze aerosols into two categories by droplet size: large and small. The large droplets contain the most virus, but fall rapidly and are rarely inhaled. The small droplets may stay aloft quite a while, but they contain only minute traces of virus. In air, much of this virus quickly becomes too dry to cause infection, leaving very few live virus particles in the air.

During the 1970s, American cold researchers were largely unable to spread rhinovirus colds by the aerosol route. A study by noted cold authority Robert Couch, M.D., at the National Institutes of Health, isolated fifteen rhinovirus cold sufferers and twelve antibody-free recipients in a room divided by wire mesh. Despite large fans to assure adequate air circulation, not one of the healthy group caught the cold. Five similar studies by prominent cold researchers Elliot Dick at the University of Wisconsin, and Jack Gwaltney, Jr., M.D., and Owen Hendley, M.D., professors of Medicine and Pediatrics respectively at the University of Virginia at Charlottesville, also showed poor transmission—0 to 8 percent. It began to look as though the tiny amount of live rhinovirus available for infection by inhalation might cause a smattering of colds here and there, but nowhere near enough to infect the average person several times each year. The question remained: How did the common cold spread?

Kissing?

University of Wisconsin researchers had ten rhinovirus cold sufferers kiss sixteen antibody-free recipients "for 1.5 minutes using the kissing technique most natural to them." One recipient (6 percent) caught the cold, a proportion not all that much greater than an adult's risk of coming down with a cold by chance. The nose, not the mouth and saliva, is the source of the vast majority of infectious rhinovirus particles, and the transferred cold may have resulted from direct nose-to-nose contact. This study suggests that casual pecks on the cheek and quick dry-lip kisses do not pose an appreciable risk. But a night of extended passionate lovemaking with substantial nose-to-nose contact might. Studies show that childless married couples transfer 30 to 40 percent of their colds. So feel free to kiss when either you or the object of your affections has an upper respiratory infection. Just don't rub noses.

Hand-to-Hand Contact?

With aerosols and kissing largely ruled out, scientists were stumped. Then, in a series of experiments from 1973 to 1978, Gwaltney and Hendley revolutionized the science of the common cold by showing that transmission could occur through hand-to-hand contact followed by self-inoculation. In a key experiment, 5 percent of healthy volunteers caught colds after brief exposure to rhinovirus-infected cough and sneeze aerosols, but a whopping 73 percent became infected after hand-to-hand contact with cold sufferers and subsequent rubbing of their noses or tear ducts. (The tear ducts in the inner corners of the eyes connect directly to the nasopharynx.)

Gwaltney and Hendley also showed that rhinoviruses can survive for several hours on the hands, in cloth handkerchiefs (but not disposable paper tissues), and on hard nonporous surfaces: counters, dishes, doorknobs, telephones, and so on. They theorized that infected individuals' hands become contaminated when they rub or blow their noses. Contaminated hands deposit live virus on everyday surfaces. Unwitting victims literally pick it up on their fingers, then inoculate themselves by rubbing their tear ducts or by touching or picking their noses.

Picking their noses? Nose picking may be universal, but when Gwaltney and Hendley first published their findings, the prestigious British medical journal, *The Lancet,* sniffed editorially that it seemed impossible anything so *gauche* could be responsible for the spread of humanity's leading illness.

Undaunted, Gwaltney and Hendley secretly observed two large groups, a class of medical students and a group of Sunday school children. These groups touched their eyes or rubbed or picked their noses quite frequently, lending credence to the direct-contact/self-inoculation theory.

"Nose picking," Gwaltney explains, "is something of an overstatement. You don't have to dig the fingers deep in there. Depositing virus at the nasal opening—for example, by simply wiping the nose—transmits infection pretty well. Ordinary nose touching, which most people do subconsciously quite frequently, is good enough. The tear duct is also an efficient route of entry for cold viruses."

Even as they championed hand-to-hand transmission with self-inoculation, Gwaltney and Hendley never said that their direct-contact route was the only way colds spread, or even the primary route of transmission. All they said was that rhinovirus colds *could* be transmitted in this manner in the laboratory. It was anyone's guess how they spread in the real world.

Nonetheless, by the early 1980s, the scientific and mass media, once wedded to the aerosol theory, decided to ignore Gwaltney's and Hendley's caveats and accept hand-to-hand transmission with self-inoculation as The Answer.

They acted prematurely.

Aerosols Reconsidered

Despite the hand-to-hand theory's impressive experimental results, it, too, came in for a good deal of criticism. Skeptics charged that the experimental transmission method was "unnatural." The subjects ground their fingers into unusually large deposits of fresh, wet nasal mucus on donor hands, then vigorously ground virus-contaminated fingers into their noses and tear ducts. The result was self-inoculation with much more virus than the typical person was likely to pick up in the real world.

A British study showed that rhinovirus was infective *only* while it remained moist, ideally in fresh nasal secretions. Mucus-dampened cloth handkerchiefs could harbor infective virus, but dry virus on household objects and surfaces—presumably the form most uninfected hands encounter—appeared unable to transmit a significant amount of infection.

Then in 1986, University of Wisconsin cold researcher Elliot Dick arranged a series of experiments to test the aerosol and hand-to-hand theories at the same time, under what he termed "reasonably natural conditions." Eight adults with experimentally induced rhinovirus colds played poker with three different groups of twelve antibody-free recipients in a closed room for twelve hours. Each five-person poker game contained two cold sufferers and three healthy volunteers grouped around a small circular table, placing them close enough for long enough to approximate household aerosol exposure. Meanwhile, the constant card playing provided ample opportunity for live virus to reach uninfected fingers and noses by the hand-to-hand route. Of the twelve recipients in each test, six wore arm braces, which prevented all hand-to-face contact; they could catch the cold only by the aerosol route. The other six were unrestrained. In the end, 67 percent of the unrestrained recipients and 56 percent of the aerosol-only group caught the cold. Hand-to-hand contact increased transmission 11 percent, but the aerosol route accounted for most of the transmission.

After one of the twelve-hour poker marathons, decks of virus-coated cards were immediately used in another twelve-hour poker marathon at identical tables involving twelve antibody-free recipients. If colds could be transmitted by direct contact, these volunteers should have become infected from playing with the virus-contaminated cards. But at the end of their card games, no live virus was recovered from any of their hands, and none of the card players caught the cold.

Could aerosols be The Answer after all? Perhaps, but Dick's "natural" card game experiments have also been criticized as "unnatural." He infected a large group of volunteers with rhinovirus, then selected as his virus donors only those with the worst coughs and sneezes. Critics insist that few people would be likely to encounter such concentrated virus-contaminated aerosols in the real world. And it was possible that some unknown chemical in the plastic card coating killed the virus.

The Latest Findings

In early 1987, both Elliot Dick and Gwaltney and Hendley presented new findings. Dick's latest experiment supports aerosol transmission; the Gwaltney/Hendley study bolsters the hand-to-hand route.

Dick arranged another of his now-famous marathon card games to track rhinovirus from sufferers' noses to their hands to cards to recipients' hands and into their noses. The donors, who had bad colds, had a great deal of live virus in their noses, but after twelve hours of card playing, most recipients showed none at their nasal openings. In the few who had virus, it was dry and not infective, bolstering Dick's view that direct contact plays a minor role in cold transmission.

Gwaltney and Hendley arranged what they called a "real-world" test of direct contact. They divided a group of fifty families with young children into two groups. The mothers in the test group were given a disinfectant and instructed to treat their hands frequently to eliminate as many virus particles as possible. The mothers in the control group were given a nondisinfecting substance with the same instructions. The study ran every September, a peak month for rhinovirus activity, for four consecutive years, 1983 through 1986. Gwaltney declined to dicuss his results in detail because at press time they had not been published in a scientific journal, but he said he is "moderately pleased," a hint that the families who used the disinfectant suffered significantly fewer colds because of interruption of direct contact.

Where do these contradictory studies leave us? Right where they leave cold researchers themselves—with as many questions as answers. "We still don't know how colds are transmitted under natural conditions," Gwaltney writes. "Owen Hendley and I have unquestionably established that rhinovirus colds can be transmitted by hand-to-hand contact with self-inoculation. Elliot Dick has unquestionably established that they can be transmitted by aerosols. It's certainly possible that both routes are important in the real world."

"In practical terms," Dick writes, "rhinovirus colds are not likely to be transmitted by either route to healthy individuals who have only brief contact with cold sufferers in most public places—stores or movie theaters. Also, stays of a few hours among those with rhinovirus colds are not likely to result in contagion, even if infected and uninfected individuals embrace briefly. Transmission is more likely when persons are exposed to cold sufferers for extended periods of time in familylike environments, or when parents soil their hands with moist nasal secretions while wiping the nose of an infected child, then inoculating themselves by touching their noses or rubbing their eyes."

Despite their continuing scientific disagreement, Jack Gwaltney and Elliot Dick enjoy cordial relations. "We've been friends for decades," Dick says. "We talk frequently, and review each other's work. We both try to keep open minds."

"Personally, I don't care which way the issue is resolved," Gwaltney says. "I just want to know the answer."

How the Other Cold Viruses Spread

So far, the discussion of cold transmission has focused exclusively on the rhinoviruses. Although they are the leading cause of colds, and the focus of most transmission research, they cause no more than half of upper respiratory infections. Cold researchers are careful to specify that their transmission studies apply only to rhinovirus colds. Unfortunately, the media often do not distinguish among the seven families of upper respiratory viruses and often mistake "rhinovirus colds" for "all colds." The fact is that the other families of cold viruses each spread in their own way, and some differ markedly from the rhinoviruses.

- Parainfluenza viruses, which account for 15 to 25 percent of colds, are spread by both aerosol and direct contact, but scientists are not sure which route is primary.
- Influenza viruses, which cause 10 to 20 percent of

upper respiratory infections (more during periodic epidemics), are spread primarily by aerosol, though direct contact with self-inoculation is also possible (see chapter 18).

• Little is known about the transmission of human coronavirus, which accounts for 10 to 20 percent of colds; however, it has been recovered from the respiratory tract and from fecal samples. Fecal/oral or fecal/nasal transmission may be possible among infants.

• Coxsackieviruses, which in combination with the echoviruses cause 5 to 10 percent of colds, are among the best aerosol-spreading cold viruses. Studies show that when antibody-free volunteers are exposed to aerosols produced by cold sufferers infected with Coxsackie-21 virus, close to 100 percent catch the cold.

• Echoviruses boast more routes of transmission than any other cold virus. They do not shed well from the respiratory tract, so the aerosol route does not seem significant. However, these viruses can be recovered from the entire digestive tract, from mouth to feces. A common contaminant of sewage, echoviruses typically survive sewage treatment and even water chlorination. They may even be spread by houseflies.

• Finally, adenoviruses, which cause 3 to 7 percent of colds, shed from the respiratory tract and in feces. Authorities suggest that fecal-oral transmission is a likely route of transmission in infants.

Remember, scientists still do not know what causes up to 25 percent of colds. These "other colds" may spread by routes not yet even discovered.

CHAPTER
6

Cold Prevention:
From "Killer Tissues"
to Selfless Love

Humorist Robert Benchley once addressed himself to the mysteries of preventing the common cold. Among his suggestions:

- Don't breath through your mouth or nose.
- Avoid crowds. Stay in your room all day with the door locked.
- Get plenty of sleep—especially at work.
- Stay in a temperature range from 60° to 70°—by lying on the sand in Palm Beach.
- Eat a balanced diet. No proteins, no starches, no carbohydrates.
- Don't stir up poisons in the body with exercise. Sit still and smoke constantly.
- Above all, don't catch colds.

No matter which virus is responsible for the week of misery most colds bring, the all-too-common cold often seems impossible to prevent. Beyond the most basic general health advice—eat right, get adequate rest and exercise, and don't smoke—the only widely practiced cold-prevention strategy is nutritional supplementation with vitamin C (see "Nutrition for Cold Prevention," below, and chapter 9).

The Susceptibility Factor

Everyone knows people who swear that ever since they started doing X, they've suffered fewer colds. X may be anything. While writing this book, your humble author was harangued by aficionados of several X factors: prune juice with breakfast each morning (good for regularity, but of no known value against colds); red wine and extra-strong garlic bread with dinner (tasty, but of little or no value against colds); and frequent phone calls to one's mother (my mother swears by this one).

Some X factors may truly work, especially if they inspire altruism (see "Selfless Love," below), or true belief (see chapter 7). But before you stock up on prune juice or whatever X factor your second cousin's brother-in-law declares freed him from colds, at least consider the possibility that the X factor may be an artifact of its promoter's changing susceptibility status. Recall that cold susceptibility decreases with age, income, and social support and increases with crowding, stress, and contact with children, particularly infants. If an overworked, underpaid nurse in a pediatrician's office who shares an apartment with three acquaintances far away from her family and close friends suddenly moves back to her hometown, takes a better-paid, less demanding job with a gerontologist, and gets a place of her own, her increased social support and decreased stress and contact with children should translate to fewer colds—even if she swears the reason is chocolate chip cookies before bed.

Vaccines: Good News . . . And Bad

Recall that hopes for a cold vaccine faded in the 1960s as the number of cold viruses climbed to its current level near two hundred. Vaccines are highly specific; most work against only one germ by stimulating the immune system to produce antibodies to the organism's unique surface proteins (antigens). As antigen variation increases, vaccine effectiveness plummets. Cold viruses have more antigen variation than any other disease organisms. In 1972, Dorland J. Davis, then a ranking official of the National Institutes of Health, told the House Appropriations Committee that the NIH was "giving up" on attempts to develop a cold vaccine.

However, recent research has produced at least a glimmer of hope that a vaccine against a manageable number of antigens might protect the public against a substantial proportion of colds. During the early 1980s, researchers at the University of Washington in Seattle studied the antibodies the various cold viruses stimulate the body to produce. They discovered that fifty of ninety cold viruses could be organized into just sixteen groups that shared significant antigen similarities. If, say, two-thirds of colds could be prevented with a single shot containing the sixteen groups of shared antigens, vaccination might prove commercially viable, especially for the elderly, the chronically ill, and others at risk for cold complications.

But just as the long-sought common-cold vaccine was being given an unexpected shot in the arm, it was largely shot down in 1985 by Purdue and University of Wisconsin biologists, who developed the first complete three-dimensional map of a rhinovirus. Purdue's Michael G. Rossman,

Ph.D., and Wisconsin's Roland R. Ruckert, Ph.D., used advanced X-ray crystallography techniques to generate fully 6 million bits of information on rhinovirus RV-14, which, ironically, is among the simplest of the cold viruses. They fed the data into a supercomputer and out came a picture of RV-14, which resembles a miniature twenty-sided soccer ball with a dent in one side, which fits over receptor areas on nasopharyngeal cells. At first it looked as though such maps might help determine the precise antigenic similarities among the various cold viruses. Then Rossman and Ruckert discovered that RV-14 (and presumably other cold viruses) is a chameleon. Its antigen sites can change without changing the virus's infectivity, a discovery that could complicate, if not cripple, vaccine development. Most scientists never say "never," but the majority of researchers call a cold vaccine "impossible."

Nutrition and Cold Prevention

Like every other part of the body, the immune system cannot function properly without adequate nutrition. The classic nutritional-deficiency diseases—malnutrition, scurvy, rickets, and so on—are virtually unheard of in the United States today. On the other hand, in a nation that smokes billions of cigarettes, abuses alcohol, takes birth control pills and many other legal and illegal drugs, guzzles soft drinks to the tune of $30 billion a year, grabs more and more fast-food meals on the run, is exposed to hundreds of pollutants, spends $10 billion a year on weight-loss programs, has one-third of its population dieting at any given moment, and embraces new—and often questionable—"miracle diets" faster than you can say "the common cold," many Americans' diets are decidedly unbalanced.

In the last few years, particularly since the AIDS epidemic has focused unprecedented attention on the immune system, several purportedly "immune-boosting" diets have been advanced, most notably the best-selling *Immune Power Diet* by Stuart M. Berger, M.D. Dr. Berger's diet certainly does no harm; in fact, as a low-fat, high-fiber diet based on whole grains, fresh fruits and vegetables, and moderate vitamin and mineral supplementation, most nutritionists would have few quarrels with it. The problem with best-selling diets—even the balanced ones—is that they demand a great deal of concentration and planning and, as a result, come and go as quickly as clothing fashions.

A less demanding, more conservative approach to maintaining a healthy immune system is to follow the guidelines of the American Heart Association (AHA) and the American Cancer Society (ACS) for the prevention of cancer, stroke, and heart disease, the nation's three leading killers. The AHA and ACS guidelines are based on a tremendous amount of laboratory and epidemiological research. They are also remarkably similar.

There is comparatively little research on dietary approaches to preventing viral infections, but the studies that have been performed support an immunity-enhancing role for fresh, whole foods rich in vitamins A, C, E, fiber, and several minerals, all of which are richly supplied by the AHA/ACS diet:

• *Eat less fat.* A high-fat diet is strongly associated with cancer, stroke, and heart disease. Substitute fish, skinned chicken, and pastas for red meats, cheeses, and eggs. Substitute yogurt for sour cream, and low- or non-fat milk for whole milk. Cut down on fried foods by steaming, broiling, or baking. Substitute fruits and sorbets for ice cream and other rich desserts.

• *Eat more high-fiber foods.* Dietary fiber protects against several cancers, and high-fiber diets tend to be low in fat. High-fiber foods include: whole-grain cereals and breads and fresh fruits and vegetables.

• *Eat foods rich in vitamins A, C, E, and the B vitamins.*

These nutrients are associated with a lower risk of cancer and a more responsive immune system. Orange and dark green vegetables are high in vitamin A. Citrus fruits and many vegetables are high in vitamin C (see chapter 9). Fresh vegetables and vegetable oils are high in vitamin E. Whole grains and fresh fruits and vegetables are also rich in the B vitamins.

• *Eat more cabbage, broccoli, cauliflower, and brussels sprouts.* These "cruciferous" vegetables have been associated with lower rates of certain cancers.

• *Eat fewer smoked, salt-cured, and nitrite-cured foods.* These contain chemical carcinogens.

• *Don't smoke.*

• *Drink alcohol in moderation, if at all.*

• *If you take vitamins, take a multivitamin and mineral "insurance formula" supplement.* Taking large quantities of single vitamins (other than vitamin C) may adversely affect the absorption of other nutritents.

"Killer Tissues"

While scientists continue to debate the major route of cold transmission, they agree that, in the words of Wisconsin cold researcher Elliot Dick, "The great majority of colds spread because of indolence. It might be possible to prevent transmission through careful personal hygiene."

Dick tested this approach at McMurdo Station, a U.S. Research station in Antarctica. "Antarctica is a great place to study colds," Dick says. "It's one of the few places on earth with a truly isolated population. About fifty Navy personnel stay through the Antarctic winter, and by spring, their colds have pretty much died out. Then about a hundred and fifty summer people arrive, and all two hundred remain isolated from the rest of the world—and from new cold viruses—for six weeks. The summer people typically bring twenty to thirty colds into McMurdo's no-colds environment. We tracked the spread of those colds from 1975 through 1978 and consistently observed a flat curve— twenty to thirty colds throughout the summer season, no epidemic outbreaks, just a steady rate of one or two new colds a day."

To test his disinfection idea, Dick impregnated Kleenex-brand facial tissues with iodine, a powerful disinfectant that kills 99.9 percent of upper respiratory viruses within one minute of contact, then returned to McMurdo for the Antarctic summer of 1979.

"We had three years of experience with a steady twenty to thirty colds at all times. When the 1979 summer group arrived, we let the usual outbreak begin. For two weeks, we observed the familiar pattern. Then we handed out the iodine-impregnated tissues. Someone called them Killer Kleenex and the name stuck. We placed them in the mess hall food line and at about thirty other high-traffic locations around the base. We also did a good deal of personnel education, and everyone used the tissues religiously. The great thing about virucidal tissues is that they disinfect the hands, face, and nasal secretions at the same time, so we had both the aerosol and direct-contact routes reasonably covered. For four days, the McMurdo population continued to have the usual twenty to thirty colds. Then suddenly, the number of colds dropped off dramatically. Ten days after the introduction of the virucidal tissues, we were down to just five colds, a seventy-five percent decrease. Treated Kleenex tissues looked miraculous."

Unfortunately, it also looked like a commercial loser. Iodine stains. By the end of the experiment, the McMurdo population all had red-brown noses and hands. Iodine also smells unpleasant and provokes allergies in some people.

But Dick's 75 percent reduction in colds was nothing to sneeze at. Dick took his "miraculous" results and his iodine problem to scientists at Kimberly-Clark, maker of Kleenex tissues, who suggested replacing the iodine with a combination of citric and malic acid to kill acid-sensitive cold viruses, and sodium lauryl sulfate, a mild detergent, to kill influenza viruses. This combination is almost as effective as iodine, without the staining, odor, or allergy problem.

In 1985, Dick tested new-and-improved virucidal Kleenex tissues at one of his mucus-soaked card games. Eight men with severe rhinovirus colds played poker for twelve hours with several groups of a dozen antibody-free recipients. In the test games, the cold sufferers used the treated tissues diligently. In the control games, the cold sufferers used ordinary cloth handkerchiefs whenever they felt like it. The results surpassed the McMurdo test. *Not one* of the recipients in the virucidal tissues group caught the cold, whereas 42 to 75 percent of those in the control groups did.

Sensing a potential commercial bonanza, Kimberly-Clark test-marketed new-formula virucidal Kleenex during the 1985–86 cold and flu season under the brand name Avert in Buffalo, Rochester, and Albany, New York. A report in *The Wall Street Journal* said that the tissues did not sell well. No one knew of Dick's stunning success with personal disinfection, and Avert tissues cost three times as much as regular Kleenex tissues. A Kimberly-Clark spokesman declined to comment on the Avert tissue test-marketing experiment, but said that the company is "optimistic" about eventually marketing a disinfecting tissue nationally.

Civilization's Infection

Ancient references to the common cold suggest that it is one of humanity's oldest ailments. But in evolutionary terms it's among the newest. Elliot Dick explains: "Unlike many other microorganisms that cause illness in a variety of species, most cold viruses infect only chimpanzees and humans. Parasites can evolve only in the presence of supportive hosts, so advanced primates had to precede the appearance of cold viruses."

Some germs can become dormant and survive for long periods outside their hosts, but not cold viruses. Outside the nasopharynx, they die fairly quickly. So where do cold viruses go when no one has a cold?

"Someone *always* has a cold," Dick says. "Our research suggests that one to five percent of the population is in some stage of infection at all times. But in our Antarctic studies, after the summer people left, colds basically died out in the small group that spent the winter. Without a 'critical mass' of people to sustain them, especially children, cold viruses can't survive. In other words, colds require relatively large numbers of people in close proximity, with new people coming and going to catch and spread them. This strongly suggests that cold viruses could not have evolved until *Homo sapiens* abandoned their small hunting and gathering groups and came together in populations large enough, with enough children, to provide a permanent reservoir of infection—in other words, until the beginnings of civilization, with trade probably a key factor in transmission."

Do-It-Yourself Disinfection

Fortunately, we can prevent many colds without resorting to quarantines or specially treated tissues. When you have a cold, or come in contact with cold sufferers:

• *Wash your hands frequently with soap and water.* Although self-inoculation may not be the primary route of viral transmission, colds can spread by direct contact. Wash your hands after using them to cover your mouth when sneezing or coughing. Also wash after shaking hands or any close contact with cold sufferers, especially children. Teach your children to do the same.

• *Keep your hands away from your nose and eyes.* Even if you contaminate your fingers with live virus, this prevents self-inoculation.

• *Use disposable facial tissues, not cloth handkerchiefs.* "Cloth handkerchiefs harbor virus," says cold researcher Jack Gwaltney. "The dampness keeps the virus infective. Every time the handkerchief is used, the hands become recontaminated. But cold viruses do not survive well in disposable tissues—even the regular untreated kind."

• *Disinfect children's toys and household and workplace objects and surfaces with Lysol.* Gwaltney and Hendley tested a variety of common disinfectants for their ability to kill cold viruses. Iodine worked best, but its problems make it impracticable. Alcohol was surprisingly ineffective. Lysol Spray proved "moderately effective." Lysol disinfection of ceramic tiles contaminated by rhinovirus reduced experimental cold transmission by 20 percent.

• *Finally, try to stay home for the first day or two of cold symptoms—when shedding peaks.* This may not be possible, but if everyone did so, and if parents kept their children home from school and day care as well, the colds "going around" would get around a lot less.

To the extent that colds can spread by the aerosol route, virus-trapping air filtration would seem to hold the most promise. Elliot Dick says that infective cold viruses are able to remain airborne when in clumps no larger than two to three microns in diameter (.00008 to .00012 inches). "We're trying to design air filtration experiments right now to remove cold viruses from the air and see if that prevents transmission." Several air filters already on the market claim to filter particles as small as .3 microns. It remains to be seen whether these devices can actually prevent the spread of colds, but they might (see the resource list at the end of this chapter).

• • •

Houseplants and Negative Air Ions

Several studies have linked low relative humidity to decreased IgA production and an increased incidence of colds. No studies show that raising relative humidity actually prevents colds, but humidification is widely recommended for treatment (see chapter 8), and the idea makes some preventive sense. Humidifying devices are one way to go, and a report in the *British Medical Journal* suggests that broad-leafed houseplants might also help. Leafy houseplants transpire significant amounts of water vapor and help maintain relative humidity above 50 percent, the level associated with a decreased risk of colds.

In addition to increasing air quality and relative humidity, houseplants—and such garden appointments as miniature waterfalls—also add negative ions to the atmosphere. Air ions are gas molecules that bear either a positive or negative charge. Formed by natural interactions among wind, land, water, plant life, and naturally occurring background radiation, fresh unpolluted air has 1,000 to 4,000 ions per cubic centimeter. Changes in the air ion balance have surprisingly significant effects on the respiratory health of laboratory animals and humans.

A predominance of positive ions or ion-depleted air is associated with fatigue, irritability, and upper respiratory problems. A predominance of negative ions or air rich in ions with a balance of positive and negative tends to enhance feelings of health and well-being. The so-called "winds of ill repute"—the Santa Ana winds of California, the sirocco in Italy, the mistral of France, and the Sharav in Israel—all deplete the air of ions and are associated with a wide range of mood and respiratory problems. On the other hand, many traditional health spas are located in areas that are naturally rich in air ions, with a predominance of negative ions.

Research by Albert P. Kreuger at the University of California at Berkeley suggests that air ions exert their effects by altering blood and brain levels of serotonin, a powerful hormone that affects many body processes. Positive ions raise serotonin levels, and negative ions lower them.

Smoking, synthetic fibers, air pollutants, VDT screens, central heating, and air conditioning all deplete air ions to the point where, at the end of a workday in a typical office, the air may contain less than 5 percent the number of ions found in fresh, unpolluted air. Studies show that both high concentrations of positive ions and ion-depleted air increase laboratory animals' death rates from respiratory diseases. And a study of two groups of employees at a Swiss bank demonstrated a significant increase in absences due to respiratory illnesses among those who worked in an ion-depleted environment compared with those whose office air was ion-enriched using a negative-ion generator (see resources).

Selfless Love

Since stress is a major factor in cold susceptibility, does stress reduction provide a protective effect? Absolutely, according to many recent studies, some of which take science into the realm of religion.

Stress reduction means "relaxation," but not the kind that involves a six-pack, an overstuffed chair, and the Game of the Week. Potentially cold-preventive stress-control regimens include: yoga, meditation, massage, biofeedback, some forms of exercise, Benson relaxation response, progressive muscle relaxation, music appreciation—even prayer.

Potentially cold-preventive forms of relaxation all involve: a conscious emptying of the mind of everyday cares and anxieties; an equally conscious channeling of emotional energy "inward" to a place of inner contentment; use of the imagination to visualize "oneness," peace, and harmony; heightened awareness of the "now"; and the realization that each of us is only a tiny part of some Greater Whole (for more on specific regimens, see resources).

Recently, meditative techniques have been shown to bolster the immune system considerably. In a study in *Psychosomatic Medicine,* researchers taught volunteers one of four relaxation techniques—massage, guided visualization, Benson relaxation response, or simply lying quietly with eyes closed focusing inward—and measured the IgA in their saliva before and after a single twenty-minute relaxation period. Each relaxation method boosted IgA secretion significantly. Control subjects, who spent the twenty minutes in a nonmeditative state completing a simple task, experienced no IgA increase. No relaxation method was significantly better than any other. The authors suggest that those interested in boosting their first line of defense against the common cold should "practice the relaxation method(s) they find most enjoyable."

In another experiment, Harvard researchers placed forty-five healthy volunteers in one of three groups. Fifteen were trained in deep breathing and progressive muscle relaxation. Another fifteen learned the same relaxation techniques and received additional instruction in guided imagery. They envisioned their T-cells attacking cold and flu viruses. The third fifteen-person group received neither relaxation nor visualization training. Before and after the relaxation/visualization training, researchers measured subjects' IgA output and number of helper T-cells. The control subjects showed no change in either immune system measurement. The "relaxers" increased their IgA levels. The "relaxer/visualizers" increased both their IgA levels and their T-cell counts.

The implication is that meditative relaxation plus some vision of self-healing helps the immune system rev up. A recent study by David C. McClelland, Ph.D., a professor of psychology at Harvard, supports this view. McClelland's studies of the immune system changes spurred by visions of healing led him to investigate people who claimed to have a spiritual healing gift. He concluded that the healers' communication of *caring,* rather than anything specific about their faith or individual healing techniques, seemed to be the crucial ingredient in any success they enjoyed.

To study the effects of this caring, McClelland measured IgA in a group of Harvard students, then screened a documentary film about Mother Teresa of Calcutta, the Nobel Prize–winning nun who works with that city's sick and poor. About half the students admired her caring and humanity. The rest disapproved of her; some even called her "a fake." But independent of what the students thought of her, *all* their IgA levels increased.

At first McClelland was surprised. He expected IgA increase to be closely correlated with viewer belief in Mother Teresa's saintliness, but it was not. Further analysis suggested that belief in the healer's personal power was not as important to IgA production as belief in his or her sincerity and altruism, which McClelland dubbed "selfless love."

Of course, it's one thing to increase IgA output and quite another to prevent real colds. So McClelland divided twenty-six students who reported early cold symptoms into two groups. One received considerable personal, sincere, altruistic attention from a self-styled evangelistic healer. He told them that they were wonderful people who possessed the power to heal themselves and exhorted them to do so. The others saw the healer only briefly and were dismissed abruptly without any personal attention and without the self-healing pep talk. In the "healed" group, eleven of the thirteen did not come down with the cold. They also showed substantial increases in IgA output. In the control group, eleven of the thirteen caught the cold and showed little change in IgA.

This research may partially explain the panreligious belief that "good works are rewarded," as well as at least some examples of "faith-healing." Altruism and acts of selfless love apparently work as "spiritual vaccines" that stimulate the immune system to cure illness. Viewed in this context, the common cold may be God's way of chastising those of little Faith and Charity.

RESOURCES

Biotech Air Purifier and Negative Ion Generator. Contains a patented filtration system that removes particles down to less than 1 micron in diameter. Also generates negative ions. Consumes no more electricity than a 100-watt light bulb and operates quietly enough for bedroom use at night. For more information, contact the *Self-Care Catalog*. The *Catalog* is free from 11 Chapel St., Augusta, Me. 04330; (207) 622-5949.

Stress Management Items. For information on meditative disciplines, biofeedback devices, relaxation cassette tapes, and massage instruction and supplies, contact the *Self-Care Catalog*, address above.

C H A P T E R

7

Cold Cure or Placebo? Not Even Your Doctor Knows for Sure

Before we delve into the many cold treatments, it's important to understand that marvelous self-care phenomenon, the placebo effect. In Latin, *placebo* means "I will please." In modern medicine, a placebo is a treatment that has no pharmacological action. Researchers use placebos to test drug effectiveness. They divide a group with a particular ailment into two subgroups. One receives the drug being tested; the other receives the trappings but not the treatment: an identical-looking pill that contains only inert ingredients like sugar or cornstarch. To be judged effective, the new drug must produce significantly greater relief than the placebo.

Such tests, however, prove a great deal more than just the effectiveness of new drugs. They also consistently show that in a surprisingly large proportion of cases, placebos *work*.

In a classic 1955 study, Henry K. Beecher, M.D., a Harvard anesthesiologist, reviewed fifteen studies involving 1,100 patients with a variety of ailments—heart disease, pain, and cold symptoms, among others—and found that on average, 35 percent of placebo takers reported significant relief. In the five studies Beecher reviewed that focused on cold remedies, 40 percent of placebo takers reported relief. Many studies over the last thirty years have confirmed Beecher's findings, so much so, in fact, that contemporary pharmacologists generally assume that placebo effects account for a significant proportion of the effectiveness of all drugs. This is certainly the case with cold remedies.

Allies

Medical researchers usually treat the placebo effect as an annoyance, a confounding variable that, if not eliminated, is certain to pollute their findings. But on a deeper level, those who view medicine as a science, as opposed to an art, often find the placebo phenomenon downright *embarrassing.* From their perspective, placebo effects simply show how gullible people are. You tell patients that a worthless pill works wonders, and it actually provides relief for a third of them, the fools.

However, from a self-care perspective, the placebo effect is an important health ally. Placebos prove that a great deal of healing is *self-healing.* It comes from within us, independent of drugs and other treatments.

How do placebos actually work? This was a mystery until 1978, when researchers linked their effects to endorphins, morphinelike substances produced by the body that act on receptors in the brain and spinal cord to reduce pain. Researchers at the University of California's San Francisco Medical Center gave fifty adults suffering pain from impacted wisdom teeth either an opiate painkiller or a placebo, both followed by naloxone, which blocks the effects of narcotics, negating their pain relief. The naloxone blocked both the opiate and the placebo, suggesting that placebos have the same effects on the body as opiates. The implication is that the user's belief in the placebo somehow stimulates the release of endorphins, the body's own natural opiates.

Enthusiasm and Belief

You don't have to be gullible to find relief from placebos, nor is there any "placebo personality." But it turns out that placebo effectiveness is associated with several contextual factors:

PROVIDER ENTHUSIASM. The "enthusiasm effect" becomes clear from a German experiment on pain. Two groups with toothaches were given the same placebo. One was told that the pill completely eliminated all pain almost immediately. The other was told that it helped some people somewhat. Guess which group experienced the pain relief? Further tests showed that the enthusiasm effect was independent of the provider's bedside manner. Placebos given by warm, empathetic physicians who exhibited no enthusiasm for them produced significantly less relief than identical placebos prescribed by cold, aloof physicians who were enthusiastic.

In a 1979 essay in the *New England Journal of Medicine,* researchers David McCallie and Herbert Benson, the Harvard professor whose "relaxation response" was mentioned in chapter 6, wrote that throughout medical history, whenever a drug or treatment has first been introduced, "there has been general enthusiasm with initial reports of 70 to 90 percent effectiveness. Only later have more adequately controlled studies appeared, performed by skeptics, in which effectiveness has decreased to 30 to 40 percent."

During the nineteenth century, the power of physician

enthusiasm was so well established that medical students learned this dictum: "Use the new drugs quickly, while they still have the power to heal."

USER BELIEF. In a 1965 experiment, experienced users of the powerful hallucinogen LSD were given a placebo but told that it was the drug. They reported typical LSD effects. Subsequently they were given real LSD but told that it was a placebo. None experienced hallucinations.

Faith in a treatment—and in one's health provider—is crucial to therapeutic success. As discussed in chapter 6, sometimes faith alone boosts IgA levels enough to prevent colds. The most powerful placebo effects result from the combination of provider enthusiasm and user belief.

SYMPTOM SEVERITY. As symptom severity increases, placebo relief also increases. Severe symptoms foster desperation, and those who feel desperate tend to be more willing to believe.

Keep the placebo effect in mind as we survey the various cold cures. The one(s) that work best for you are likely to be the ones you trust the most. Physicians often dismiss alternative cold remedies—vitamin C, herbs, hot toddies, and so on—as "mere placebos." But as we shall see, a substantial body of research suggests that some of the cold remedies most widely recommended by doctors, particularly antihistamines, owe a good deal of their effectiveness to the placebo effect, as well.

Over-the-Counter Cold Remedies

There's an old saying that if left untreated, colds last a week, but when treated aggressively, they clear up in just seven days.

Such fatalism is understandable. Despite the immune boost of the placebo effect, many cold remedies don't produce much relief. But even hardened cynics rarely leave their colds untreated. Ironically, most people who use commercial cold formulas *overtreat* themselves and might recover faster—at lower cost—if they did less.

According to orthodox medicine, there is no cure for the common cold. Although practitioners of alternative healing arts would disagree, this chapter presents the standard medical view, which holds that the only real cure is time. Over a week or so, the immune system attacks, contains, and finally defeats the cold virus. In the meantime, orthodox medicine's goal is "symptomatic relief," alleviation of discomfort until the body heals itself.

The vast majority of colds may be treated safely at home without consulting a health professional. However, good self-care involves recognizing situations that call for a physician. Those over age seventy, or under ten, or those who are pregnant or nursing, or who have heart disease, asthma, emphysema, diabetes, serious allergies, liver or kidney disease, a history of stroke, or other significant health problems should consult a physician before using the remedies discussed here and in the following chapters. Even if you're healthy, it's crucial to understand the effects and potential side effects of any cold medications you use.

Multisymptom Formulas Versus Single-Symptom Generics

When colds strike, millions of Americans immediately reach for one of the heavily advertised, multisymptom cold formulas. Americans spend more than $1 billion a year on these products, but *none* of the cold researchers or clinical authorities consulted for this book recommended them—including the Food and Drug Administration's (FDA) 1976 Advisory Review Panel on Over-the-Counter (OTC) Cold, Cough, and Allergy Products. The experts unanimously recommend single-symptom generic drugs. Single-action generics cost much less and pose no risk of side effects from extra drugs that are unnecessary for the specific symptoms cold sufferers have at any given time.

From an advertising perspective, there's an undeniable allure to the claim that a cold formula "treats every major symptom." But cold symptoms appear serially, not all at once: first the odd feeling that a cold is coming on; then the sore throat; followed by the malaise, lethargy, and possibly fever and body aches; then the runny nose and nasal congestion; and finally the cough. By treating every cold symptom at once, consumers automatically pay extra for medication they don't need and risk side effects from the superfluous ingredients. In addition, these products may not contain enough of the specific medication(s) necessary to relieve one's symptoms at any particular time. Finally, most shotgun cold formulas contain ingredients that have no effect whatsoever on cold symptoms, for example caffeine (see "Hidden Ingredients," below), which may also cause adverse effects. Cold authorities urge consumers to take maximum control of their self-treatment through judicious use of single-action OTCs to treat individual symptoms as they occur.

Single-symptom OTCs—especially generic drugs sold under their chemical names instead of the more familiar brand names—save a great deal of money. The cost of advertising a multisymptom cold formula is incorporated into its price. Today it's easier than ever to buy generic drugs, as pure and effective as their brand-name counterparts, for *25 to 90 percent less.* Just ask your pharmacist for the single-action generics discussed throughout this chapter.

Although I generally agree with consumer advocates who say it's silly to spend up to ten times extra simply to support TV commercials for multisymptom cold formulas, on the other hand, brand-name advertising just might play a role in the products' effectiveness. Recall that provider enthusiasm and user belief are key elements in the self-healing placebo effect. There are no studies to show that glitzy commercials and slick advertisements are as immune-boosting as physician enthusiasm, but this certainly seems possible. Ads for multisymptom cold remedies are everywhere, and most consumers hear them much more frequently than they hear their physicians wax enthusiastic about anything. The actors in cold-formula ads uniformly experience fast, Fast, FAST relief. In just sixty seconds, their symptoms vanish. Consumer advocates attack cold-formula advertising as misleading. On the one hand, it is. But on the other, who knows? If physician enthusiasm can increase a drug's effectiveness, perhaps a hard sell can, too. Personally, I'd still recommend lower-priced, single-action alternatives, but if, after trying some generics, you honestly believe that a brand-name cold formula is worth the extra money, there's no reason not to use it.

Whether you use generics or brand-name remedies, you're buying the same medications, approved and regulated identically by the FDA. However, FDA approval in no way implies government endorsement. All it means is that the product has been judged safe and *possibly* effective at the dosage specified on the package.

Cold-medication "effectiveness" is a matter of sometimes passionately divided opinion. Some FDA-approved cold remedies—dextromethorphan for cough, for example—are backed by unassailable evidence of effectiveness. But others—for example, antihistamines—are surprisingly controversial; they may or may not be effective (see below). FDA approval hinges more on safety than effectiveness.

Any cold symptom might signal an illness more serious than the common cold. OTC cold remedies should not be used more frequently or at higher doses than their packaging indicates. Seek professional help if you develop any of the symptoms discussed in the section "Rx: What Doctors—and Grandmothers—Recommend Most," or in chapters 17 and 18.

Read Labels

Many people are intimidated by the long chemical names of the drugs in OTC cold medications. Brand-name remedies were developed in part to simplify drug selection.

But they often confuse matters further—and always add to cost. Different brand-name formulas may contain virtually identical ingredients, and even if some ingredients are chemically different, their action is often the same. To know what you're getting, it's crucial to read labels. For example, here are the active ingredients in four popular cold remedies:

Dristan
phenylephrine
  hydrochloride
chlorpheniramine maleate
acetaminophen

Contac
phenylpropanolamine
chlorpheniramine maleate
acetaminophen

Comtrex
phenylpropanolamine
chlorpheniramine maleate
acetaminophen
dextromethorphan

Nyquil
pseudoephedrine
doxylamine succinate
acetaminophen
dextromethorphan
alcohol (25%)

At first glance, it may seem difficult to make sense of these tongue twisters, but actually it's fairly easy. The first ingredient in each is a decongestant; the second, an antihistamine; and the third, a painkiller. Comtrex and Nyquil also contain a fourth, a cough suppressant. And Nyquil, like virtually all liquid cold formulas, contains a good deal of alcohol.

Brand-name cold formulas come and go, but their ingredients remain the same. That's why this chapter focuses on the chemical names of the various ingredients. Once you're familiar with them, it's easy to understand the combinations that turn up in the fine print on labels of any "new" remedies "doctors recommend most."

Sore-Throat Remedies

Packaged as lozenges, gargles, or sprays, sore-throat remedies provide temporary relief of minor pain. They do not kill cold viruses or speed healing. FDA-approved sore-throat remedies are not recommended for more than two days of continuous use. If pain persists or becomes more severe, consult a physician. Although most sore-throat remedies rarely cause adverse reactions—usually allergies—a few (for example, phenol) may prove toxic at unusually high doses.

Several anesthetics have proven safe and effective for cold-related sore throat:

- Benzocaine
- Dyclonine hydrochloride
- Salicyl alcohol
- Benzyl alcohol
- Hexylresorcinol
- Phenol (sodium phenolate)

In lozenges, these drugs typically begin to work within one to five minutes and provide relief for ten to thirty minutes. They may be taken every two hours.

Aspirin, which relieves inflammation, may also help (see below). Several FDA-approved traditional herbal sore-throat remedies are discussed in chapter 11.

Drugs for Fever, Headache, and Body Aches

Collectively known as analgesics, the FDA has approved:

- Aspirin
- Ibuprofen
- Acetaminophen

ASPIRIN. Available as a generic, or as Bayer, or under such brand names as Anacin (aspirin and caffeine), more than 20 billion doses of aspirin are consumed in the United States each year—100 tablets per person. Aspirin is a powerful drug for relief of fever, inflammation, and aches and pains. Nonpregnant, nonnursing adults may take one or two standard tablets every four hours. Do not take more than 4,000 milligrams per day for more than ten days without consulting a physician. Aspirin is relatively safe, but it has quite a few potential side effects.

Many people have aspirin-sensitive stomachs. Stomach upset may be controlled by taking buffered aspirin (generic or Bufferin), by taking an antacid with the aspirin or by taking the drug after eating. If stomach upset persists, switch to acetaminophen. People with ulcers or gastrointestinal bleeding should not use aspirin.

Even if you experience no stomach upset, beware of aspirin overdose. The most common sign is ringing in the ears (tinnitus), which develops in some people at relatively low doses. If tinnitus develops, discontinue the drug. Aspirin-induced tinnitus usually subsides within a day, but it may persist for up to a month.

Aspirin interferes with blood clotting. Those with clotting disorders should not use it. (Some evidence suggests that aspirin's anticlotting action may help prevent heart attacks.) Extended use may also contribute to iron-deficiency anemia. High doses may interfere with liver function, a potential problem for those with liver disease or a history of alcoholism.

Allergic reactions are also possible: rash, hives, and asthma attacks. Potentially fatal allergic reactions (anaphylactic shock) are rare but possible. Asthma sufferers are at greatest risk and should check with their physicians about taking aspirin.

Aspirin *should not* be taken by pregnant women. It is

associated with an increased risk of birth defects (see chapter 15).

Finally, aspirin *should not be given to children under eighteen for colds, flu, or chicken pox.* It is associated with an increased risk of Reye's syndrome, a rare but potentially fatal condition that affects the brain and liver. Children should be given acetaminophen instead (see chapter 16).

ACETAMINOPHEN. Available as a generic (Apap or Apanol), but better known by its brand names (Tylenol, Datril, Panadol), acetaminophen is safe for nonpregnant, nonnursing adults in doses of one or two standard tablets every four hours. Like aspirin, do not take more than 4,000 milligrams per day for ten days without consulting a physician. Unlike aspirin, acetaminophen does not cause stomach upset or gastrointestinal bleeding. Large doses may, however, cause liver damage, especially in combination with alcohol. Those with liver disease or a history of alcoholism should consult their physicians. Allergic reactions are possible but rare.

IBUPROFEN. This is the pain reliever in Advil, Nuprin, Haltran, Medipren, and the prescription analgesic, Motrin. Nonpregnant, nonnursing adults may take one 200-milligram tablet every four hours. Those who are allergic to aspirin should avoid this drug. Possible side effects include rash, itching, hives, tinnitus, and stomach upset. Ibuprofen is the most expensive analgesic.

No matter which analgesic you use, if you have a fever, be sure to drink plenty of fluids—eight ounces every two hours. The excess perspiration associated with fever may cause dehydration, especially in children and the elderly. The body is more than 75 percent water, and all organ systems require adequate hydration to function properly.

Antihistamines for Runny Nose

Antihistamines were developed in France during World War II, and by the late 1940s had been hailed as wonder drugs for relief of the runny nose, itchy eyes, and nasal congestion of allergies. Several studies at that time suggested that they also relieved cold symptoms, and pharmaceutical companies quickly marketed OTC antihistamines for upper respiratory infections. But almost immediately, other studies showed that antihistamines had no effect on cold symptoms. In 1951, scientists at the Common Cold Research Unit in England denounced antihistamines as "valueless . . . having no benefit at all." The controversy has continued ever since, though you'd never know it from cold-remedy advertising or from talking to most physicians.

Thirty studies have investigated the issue since 1947. Nineteen concluded that antihistamines provide significant relief of cold-related runny nose; eleven showed they have no value beyond a placebo effect. However, according to an in-depth review by Johns Hopkins researchers, the most rigorous eight studies were evenly divided. Half supported antihistamines; half did not. The FDA Review Panel was not impressed with the evidence in favor of antihistamines and concluded, "There are insufficient data to establish the effectiveness of antihistamines in relieving symptoms of the common cold."

But if, as discussed in chapter 3, cold-infected nasopharyngeal cells release histamine, which boosts mucus production to help flush out virus particles, then why do so many studies show that antihistamines, which block this effect, fail to dry runny noses? Because histamine is only one of several mucus-stimulating factors. In the case of hay fever, there is neither infection nor inflammation, just a release of histamine, which antihistamines suppress, hence their proven effectiveness for allergies. But during a cold, independent of histamine release, inflammation and the interferons contribute to mucus production and runny nose. The upshot is that depending on the individual cold sufferer, antihistamine action may or may not dry a runny nose.

Why, then, are antihistamines so widely recommended by physicians? The Johns Hopkins researchers considered this issue in the journal *Pediatrics:* "Although antihistamines have not been proven effective for cold symptoms, there is a large patient demand for some form of physician intervention. Antihistamines are fairly innocuous drugs. Prescribing them is an understandable choice for harried physicians." In other words, they're good placebos.

OTC antihistamines are considered safe, but they are not "fairly innocuous." They are associated with an increased risk of birth defects in laboratory animals and should not be used by pregnant women. They also cause drowsiness. Users should not drive, drink alcohol, or operate machinery while taking them. Yet millions of cold sufferers take antihistamines and blithely drive as usual. Alcohol aggravates the drowsiness effect.

Fortunately, some OTC antihistamines cause less drowsiness than others:

- *Low risk of drowsiness:* chlorpheniramine maleate (Chlor-Trimeton), brompheniramine maleate, and pheniramine maleate.
- *Moderate risk:* pyrilamine maleate, thonzylamine hydrochloride, and tripelannamine hydrochloride.
- *High risk:* diphenhydramine hydrochloride (Benadryl), doxylamine succinate, and phenyltoloxamine citrate.

In some people, the caffeine or decongestants in multisymptom cold formulas compensate for any drowsiness.

Possible side effects include dry mouth, nervousness, and paradoxically, in some cases, insomnia. Those with glaucoma or prostate problems should consult a physician before taking antihistamines.

Anticholinergics for Runny Nose

Anticholinergics relieve runny nose and watery eyes by blocking the secretion of tears and nasal mucus. They also inhibit the production of saliva, sweat, and urine, and they dry bronchial secretions, making them stickier and more difficult to cough up. Those with heart disease, urinary problems, and chronic respiratory diseases should not take them.

The anticholinergics are extremely potent and should be used with caution, if at all. The FDA may ban them from OTC cold formulas, and most manufacturers have already removed them from their products.

The FDA Panel judged two of these drugs—belladonna and atropine sulfate—safe in the small doses used in OTCs, but only possibly effective.

Decongestants for Nasal Congestion

Decongestants relieve nasal stuffiness and improve breathing. They don't dry up nasal secretions; rather they constrict infection-swollen capillaries in the nasopharynx and sinuses.

Unlike antihistamines, decongestants are unquestionably effective. But they, too, have problems. Decongestants are available either topically in drops or sprays, or orally in pills or liquids. The topical forms frequently cause "rebound congestion." Topical decongestants cause the tiny muscles in the nasopharynx to contract, constricting the swollen capillaries that cause congestion. But after about three days of being forced to remain contracted by decongestant sprays, these muscles become fatigued, stop responding, and become *more swollen* than they were to begin with. For this reason, some authorities call decongestant nasal sprays "addictive": The more you use them, the more you feel you need them. If you use a topical decongestant, use it only occasionally and not for more than three consecutive days.

Those who use decongestant drops or sprays should not share applicators or spray bottles. The nose pieces provide a direct-contact route of transmission for cold viruses.

Oral decongestants don't cause rebound congestion because they reach the nasopharynx through the bloodstream in comparatively low concentrations. However, they often cause insomnia. The antihistamines in cold formulas may compensate for this effect.

The blood-vessel-constricting activity of oral decongestants may also raise blood pressure. Chronically high blood pressure (hypertension) is a key risk factor for heart disease and stroke, the top two causes of death in the United States. Those with hypertension, heart disease, or a history of stroke should not use oral decongestants. In addition, people with other significant risk factors for heart disease— diabetes, high blood cholesterol, obesity, or smoking—should consult a physician before self-medicating with oral decongestants. Those taking any of the antidepressant drugs known as MAO inhibitors (Marplan, Nardil, Parnate, Eutonyl) should also avoid oral decongestants. Finally, a recent study suggests that women trying to become pregnant should not use oral decongestants because they interfere with the secretion of cervical mucus, which assists the sperm's passage toward the egg.

Topical decongestants the FDA Review Panel judged safe and effective include:

- Ephedrine
- Ephedrine sulfate
- Propylhexedrine
- Xylometazoline
- Naphazoline hydrochloride
- Ephedrine hydrochloride
- Racephedrine hydrochloride
- Oxymetazoline hydrochloride
- Phenylephrine hydrocloride

Phenylephrine and naphazoline are the most likely to cause rebound congestion, possibly after just a few applications.

FDA-approved oral decongestants include:

- Ephedrine
- Pseudoephedrine
- Phenylephrine hydrochloride
- Phenylpropanolamine

Ephedrine, the world's oldest cold remedy, tends to cause more insomnia, nervousness, and tension than its laboratory analogue, pseudoephedrine, which has largely taken its place in OTC cold formulas. Phenylpropanolamine, quite common in OTC cold formulas, is also widely used as an appetite suppressant in OTC diet pills. Since high doses of phenylpropanolamine raise blood pressure, those who use this drug as a diet aid should not use it simultaneously to relieve congestion.

FDA-approved herbal decongestants are discussed in chapter 11.

Cough Medicines

The FDA has approved two kinds: cough suppressants (antitussives), which inhibit the brain's cough center, and expectorants, which manufacturers claim liquefy and loosen mucus, making it easier to cough up.

Cough suppressants help relieve the dry, irritating coughs that often develop toward the end of colds, but should not be used for more than a week. Cough suppressants *should not* be used for "productive" coughs, which bring up phlegm. Productive coughs help clear the respiratory tract of mucus, which may cause problems if it settles into the bronchi or lungs. Those with asthma, emphysema, smoker's cough, or other chronic respiratory conditions should also avoid cough suppressants.

FDA-approved cough suppressants include:

- Dextromethorphan
- Diphenydramine hydrochloride
- Codeine

Cough suppressants come in lozenges and liquids. Codeine cough preparations require a prescription. Possible side effects include constipation, headache, nausea, vomiting, and possibly addiction if taken for extended periods. The adult dose is 10 to 20 milligrams every four to six hours, not to exceed 120 milligrams per day.

Because codeine requires a prescription, most widely advertised OTC cough formulas contain dextromethorphan, a nonnarcotic, nonaddictive morphine derivative. Its major side effect, drowsiness, is exacerbated by alcohol. Those taking this drug should not drive, drink alcohol, or operate machinery. Beware of cold formulas that contain both an antihistamine and dextromethorphan, since both cause drowsiness. Diphenhydramine also causes drowsiness and carries the same warnings. FDA-approved herbal cough remedies are discussed in chapter 11.

The FDA Panel judged no expectorant as effective, but approved the following as safe:

- Guaifenesin
- Terpin hydrate
- Ammonium chloride
- Glyceryl guaiacolate
- Ipecac

Terpin hydrate causes nausea and vomiting in some people and may be formulated into liquids with very high alcohol content, a potential problem for those with liver disease or operators of cars or other machinery. In overdose, ipecac is a powerful inducer of vomiting. Ammonium chloride may also cause nausea and vomiting. FDA-approved herbal expectorants are discussed in chapter 11.

Beware of the many cough medicines that contain both an expectorant (typically guaifenesin or terpin hydrate) and a cough supressant (codeine or dextromethorphan). This is an irrational drug combination. The expectorant is supposed to make respiratory mucus easier to cough up; the cough suppressant stops coughing. Any loosened mucus falls into the lower respiratory tract, possibly contributing to bronchitis.

Products with both an expectorant and an anticholinergic are also irrational. The former is supposed to liquefy and loosen bronchial secretions; the latter dries and thickens them.

Hidden Ingredients

A surprisingly large proportion of multisymptom cold pills contains caffeine. This powerful addictive stimulant, found in coffee, black teas, cocoa, chocolate, and many soft drinks, has no effect whatsoever on cold viruses. Manufacturers include it in cold formulas for three reasons: to counteract the lethargy caused by colds; to counteract the drowsiness associated with antihistamines; and to replace the caffeine in coffee, which many cold sufferers find unappealing while ill, thus "preventing" the headache that is the major symptom of caffeine withdrawal.

For most people, there is nothing wrong with caffeine in moderation, *if* you know you're ingesting it. Unfortunately, many cold sufferers have no idea that they're taking this drug. In addition to contributing to insomnia, caffeine causes nervousness and anxiety and interferes with the relaxation skills that help mobilize the immune system against cold infection. It also raises blood pressure. Those with heart disease, high blood pressure, diabetes, or a history of stroke should be very aware of their caffeine consumption. Some evidence also suggests that caffeine may be associated with fibrocystic breasts, a common, often painful condition in women.

Many liquid cold formulas contain a surprisingly large amount of alcohol. Some are as much as *80 proof,* the equivalent of gin, vodka, or Scotch. Alcohol is the world's most abused drug. It has no effect whatsoever on cold viruses. However, it has been used to treat colds (and many other illnesses) for centuries. It's one thing to make a conscious choice to use alcohol as a cold remedy (see chapter 10), but quite another to take it unwittingly in liquid cold formulas. Those who are obese or have heart disease, diabetes, hypertension, a history of alcoholism, stroke, or other chronic illnesses should avoid it.

In addition, large doses of alcohol do not mix well with many other drugs used to treat the common cold. The combination of alcohol and large doses of acetaminophen may cause liver damage. Alcohol plus aspirin can cause bleeding of the stomach wall. And alcohol exacerbates the sedative effect of antihistamines, making this combination and driving especially hazardous.

Working Against the Immune System

No matter whether your cold remedies are economical single-action generics or the pricey formulas touted on TV, to the extent that they work at all, most OTCs (and some folk and herbal remedies as well) achieve their effects by interfering with the immune system's battle against the viral invasion.

Recall from chapter 2 that cold symptoms are produced not by the cold virus, but by the immune system's fight against it. Cold symptoms are part of the healing process. No studies show that taking cold remedies significantly prolongs colds, but given their effects on the immune system, that might well be the case.

Aspirin, acetaminophen, and ibuprofen all reduce fever. But during a cold, the immune system releases interleukin-1, which stimulates the brain to raise body temperature.

Fever impairs viral replication and stimulates greater T-cell and B-cell activity. Analgesics also reduce inflammation, but nasopharyngeal inflammation is one of the body's first defenses against cold infection. A study in the *Journal of the American Medical Association* shows that aspirin reduces white blood cell migration to the infected nasopharynx and suppresses release of interferons. Aspirin treatment did not prolong the colds in this study, but it significantly increased viral shedding, raising the possibility of increased cold transmission. The authors conclude that those who take aspirin for colds may be "epidemiologic hazards . . . perhaps enhancing the spread of the virus."

Similarly, antihistamines may dry a runny nose in some people, but mucus secretion helps flush virus particles and cell debris out of the infected area and keeps additional virus particles away from infected tissues.

Decongestants help clear blocked nasal passages, but they do it by vasoconstriction, reducing blood flow to the nose and throat. Unless you're so stuffed up that you can't breathe, you *want* increased blood flow. It warms the infected area and brings virus-fighting neutrophils, macrophages, T-cells, B-cells, and complement proteins to combat the virus.

Finally, caffeine may counteract the lethargy of colds, but there's a message in that symptom: Rest allows the body to focus its best energies on fighting the cold.

Rx: What Doctors—and Grandmothers—Recommend Most

Because of the immunosuppressive action of many cold medications, experts on upper respiratory infections urge cold sufferers to use *as few OTCs as possible.* In fact, the more scientists learn about the common cold, the more it appears that Grandma was right. In 1984, Kaiser-Permanente, the nation's largest health maintenance organization, consulted experts on colds and flu at several leading medical centers. Here is their advice for self-treatment:

• *Rest.* Grandma was right when she said, "Rest." The effort required to fight a cold, especially during the first few days, is the equivalent of hard physical labor, which is why colds cause lethargy. Take it easy. If possible, stay home for a day or two. In most cases, there's no need to get into bed, but rest helps spur self-healing. It also isolates cold sufferers from the uninfected, which limits transmission.

• *Bundle up.* Another of Grandma's classic recommendations, bundling up helps alleviate the chills associated with fever.

• *If you smoke, stop.* Smoking irritates the inflamed nasopharynx, depresses blood levels of vitamin C, and paralyzes the respiratory cilia, which move mucus out of the infected area. Impaired cilia mean that mucus falls into the lower respiratory tract, increasing the risk of complications.

• *Drink eight ounces of hot liquids every two hours.* Hot fluids soothe an irritated throat, help relieve nasal congestion, and prevent dehydration. Don't drink cold beverages. One study shows that they impede the movement of nasal mucus and contribute to congestion (see chapter 10).

• *For sore throat, gargle with warm salt water, suck on hard candies, and increase relative humidity.* The recommended salt mixture is one half teaspoon per eight ounces. Any hard candies may help, but if you'd like extra pain relief, look for lozenges that contain the FDA-approved anesthetics discussed in the "Sore Throat" section of this chapter. Humidify your immediate surroundings with a hot bath or shower, by inhaling steam, or with a vaporizer or humidifier (see resource). Consult a physician if swallowing becomes a problem or if you have a sore throat and a fever over 101° F with no other cold symptoms; this might be strep throat (see chapter 18).

• *For fever, headaches, and body aches, try a cool cloth on the forehead or use acetaminophen or ibuprofen.* Avoid aspirin, which increases viral shedding. Ask your pharmacist for generic acetaminophen or ibuprofen, or buy the least-expensive single-ingredient brand. Be sure to drink plenty of fluids. Seek professional help for fevers above 101° F; fevers above 100° that last more than two days; or any fever with rash, stiff neck, severe headache, and /or marked irritability or confusion—this might be meningitis, a potentially fatal condition of the fluid surrounding the brain and spinal column (see chapters 17 and 18).

• *For nasal congestion, drink hot fluids, or try a vaporizer, hot bath, or shower. At night use extra pillows to elevate the head.* If you must take something, use an FDA-approved single-action decongestant, unless you're pregnant or nursing or have any of the conditions discussed in the "Decongestant" section, in which case consult your physician. Possible side effects include: insomnia, nervousness, heart palpitations, and elevated blood pressure. Ask your pharmacist for a generic decongestant or buy the least-expensive single-ingredient brand.

• *For runny nose, use disposable tissues.* Cold viruses cannot survive long in paper tissues. But cloth handkerchiefs harbor live virus and recontaminate the fingers with virus each time they are used. Wash your hands after blowing your nose or after wiping a child's nose. If you must take something, and you're convinced that antihistamines help you, take a single-action product that contains an FDA-approved ingredient—preferably one with a low risk of drowsiness—unless you're pregnant, nursing or have any of the conditions discussed in the "Antihistamine" section, in which case, consult your physician. Possible side effects include dry mouth and drowsiness, which is exacerbated by alcohol. Ask your pharmacist for a generic antihistamine or buy the least-expensive single-ingredient brand.

• *Do not suppress productive coughs. For dry coughs, use a vaporizer, take hot showers, suck on hard candies, or ask your pharmacist for the least-expensive OTC with dextromethorphan.* Consult a physician if a productive cough brings up brown or bloody sputum; if a dry cough lasts more than two weeks; or if any cough is accompanied by fever, chills, chest pain, wheezing, or shortness of breath. These symptoms might indicate pneumonia (see chapters 17 and 18).

• *Antibiotics are powerless against colds.* Penicillin and the myriad of other antibiotics kill bacteria, but not cold viruses. Nonetheless, many people demand antibiotics for colds, and get upset with physicians who refuse to prescribe them. Antibiotics are useful *only* in the small proportion of colds that become complicated by other problems (see chapter 17). Antibiotics might stimulate a self-healing placebo effect against colds, but this is a bad idea. Use of antibiotics to treat viral illnesses may contribute to the development of hard-to-treat, antibiotic-resistant bacteria.

• *Avoid time-release medications.* Time-release pills may seem more convenient, but studies show that the reality falls far short of the advertising promise. The medication is not released uniformly. You may get too much for a while, then too little. It's better to take shorter-acting drugs more frequently.

RESOURCE

Ultrasonic Humidifier. Uses inaudible sound waves to atomize water into a fine, soothing mist. Capacity: 16 fluid ounces per hour. For information, contact the *Self-Care Catalog,* 11 Chapel St., Augusta, Me. 04330; (207) 622-5949.

9

The Vitamin C Controversy

It's difficult to recall a time when vitamin C was not the nation's most popular—and most hotly debated—cold cure. I use the word *cure* here because proponents of vitamin C insist that it has curative powers. Millions of Americans routinely take up to several grams a day, in part to prevent colds. And from the first sign of a sore throat, millions more take up to 20 grams a day throughout their colds in the belief that ascorbic acid, the vitamin's chemical name, either cures them or significantly hastens their recovery. But America's love affair with vitamin C—and the passionate controversy surrounding its use for colds—is actually less than twenty years old. It dates from the 1970 publication of *Vitamin C and the Common Cold* by Linus Pauling.

Pauling is one of the nation's most distinguished scientists. He has won two Nobel Prizes—the first, in chemistry in 1954 for his work on chemical bonding, and the second, the 1962 Peace Prize, for his leadership in opposing atmospheric nuclear weapons testing. An interest in biochemistry led him to study vitamins in the 1960s.

The original edition of *Vitamin C and the Common Cold* analyzed more than two dozen studies from the 1930s through the 1960s, which suggested that 1,000 to 20,000 milligrams of vitamin C each day (compared with the U.S. Recommended Daily Allowance of 60 milligrams) could prevent colds altogether or, failing that, reduce their duration by an average of 30 percent.

The book took America by storm. The combination of Pauling's stature and his evidence that humanity's leading illness might be substantially controlled by the same readily available vitamin that had cured scurvy two hundred years earlier triggered runs on vitamin C at drugstores, supermarkets, and natural food stores from Bangor to San Diego. Today vitamin C is by far the most popular food supplement. Thirty percent of Americans take vitamins regularly, according to a 1982 Gallup survey, and 90 percent of them—some 70 million people—take vitamin C.

But as Pauling toured the talk shows touting his cold cure, vitamin C was denounced by leading physicians and medical organizations. Dr. Charles C. Edwards, then chief of the Food and Drug Administration, called Pauling's vitamin C regimen "ridiculous." Edwards told reporters: "There have never been any meaningful scientific studies indicating that ascorbic acid is capable of preventing or curing colds."

Since 1970, during which time Pauling's now-classic book has been revised several times, the debate has intensified. Many pro and con studies have been published. On the "pro" side, a 1974 study in the prestigious *New England Journal of Medicine* reported that vitamin C treatment resulted in "30 percent fewer days of symptoms from respiratory illness . . . a significantly beneficial effect." In 1977,

Brazilian researchers documented a 50 percent reduction in colds' duration with a regimen of 6,000 milligrams per day. In 1981, Australian scientists concluded that colds treated with vitamin C had "significantly shorter average duration." And a series of experiments from 1972 through 1975 prompted Canadian researchers to write, "There is now little doubt that vitamin C reduces [cold symptoms]."

However, on the "con" side, a 1983 review of thirty-five studies, while noting that vitamin C "enhances immune responsiveness," concluded that it has "no significant benefit against colds." In a 1975 analysis in the *American Journal of Medicine,* another reviewer sniffed, "The very minor potential benefit that might result from taking ascorbic acid is not worth either the effort or the risk." The authors of the provitamin study in the *New England Journal of Medicine* previously cited conducted another experiment, which changed their minds, and in 1976 wrote, "We do not believe that vitamin C is useful as a cold remedy." Finally, in a 1986 column entitled "Vitamin Myths," *Consumer Reports* declared, "Over the past decade, 16 double-blind studies [of vitamin C as a cold remedy] have shown no benefit."

The Long Road to "Limeys"

Vitamin C became famous—and controversial—long before its association with the common cold, in fact, more than 100 years before it was chemically isolated. In 1753 in his *Treatise on Scurvy,* British naval physician James Lind claimed that citrus fruits prevented and cured the scourge of the Age of Exploration. By Lind's time, scurvy—marked by exhaustion, muscle pains, loss of teeth, hemorrhages, and severe diarrhea—had already plagued sailors for 250 years, killing thousands. Schoolchildren learn that Portuguese explorer Vasco da Gama discovered the sea route from Europe to India by sailing around Africa in 1498. But few know that during his year-long voyage, scurvy claimed the lives of 100 of his 160 crewmen. Typically, half the sailors on extended voyages to the New World succumbed, and it was by no means rare during the sixteenth and seventeenth centuries for ships to be sighted adrift on the high seas, their *entire crews* dead from scurvy.

French explorer Jacques Cartier was the first European to report a successful treatment. In 1536 after discovering Canada's Saint Lawrence River, he sailed inland to the site of present-day Quebec, where he and his crew dug in for the winter. Within a few months twenty-five men had died of scurvy and many others were gravely ill. An Indian introduced the group to a tea made from the bark and leaves of the yellow cedar tree (*Thuja occidentalis*), later shown to contain considerable vitamin C. Cartier's men recovered. But superstitions, communications problems, wars among the Eurpoean powers, and strange tales of other cures that didn't work prevented further investigation of Cartier's scurvy treatment.

Then in 1747 James Lind divided twelve scurvy sufferers into six pairs and placed them all on identical diets, except that he gave each pair one of the many reputed scurvy cures touted in sailors' lore: cider, vinegar, seawater, oranges and lemons, a drug mixture, and dilute sulfuric acid. After six days, ten of the twelve men were worse, but the two citrus eaters had completely recovered. In his *Treatise,* Lind advocated citrus rations for all seamen to control the dread disease.

Lind's recommendation was met with the same official hostility Linus Pauling has endured. Other British naval physicians, who gave sailors a syrup made from boiled citrus juices (not knowing that heat destroys vitamin C), pronounced Lind's theory worthless. Others criticized Lind when additional foods he did not test—particularly sauerkraut (also high in vitamin C)—turned out to control scurvy.

But Lind had influential partisans, chief among them Captain James Cook, discoverer of Hawaii, who carried citrus fruits and sauerkraut on his voyages and ordered his men to forage for fresh fruits and vegetables wherever they landed. During twelve years at sea, from 1768 to 1780, Cook never lost a man to scurvy.

Cook and many other British naval officers urged their superiors to require fresh fruits and vegetables to prevent scurvy, but it took until 1795, fully forty-eight years after Lind's experiment, for the Admiralty to require a daily ration of fresh lime juice—hence the term *limeys* for British sailors. Scurvy quickly ceased to be a problem for the British navy, but it continued to plague the British merchant fleet for another seventy years, until 1865, when the British Board of Trade finally required all freighters to provide lime juice.

Partisans of vitamin C's cold-curative powers are quick to draw parallels between Lind's experience and Pauling's. Lind was initially denounced but ultimately won vindication, and they predict the same for Pauling.

Of course, vitamin C's eventual acceptance as the cure for scurvy does not necessarily mean that it is destined to win equal acceptance as a cold cure. The research is contradictory. But beyond that, since the rise of pharmaceuticals, orthodox medicine has had significant blind spots in the areas of nutrition and preventive medicine. Physicians are taught to treat illness, not prevent it. Few medical schools provide more than a cursory survey of nutrition. Vitamin supplementation, in particular, seems to elicit derision from many M.D.'s—despite the fact that the American Cancer Society now urges Americans to eat foods rich in vitamins A, C, and E to help prevent cancer. To be sure, an increasing number of physicians promote sound nutrition and dietary approaches to illness prevention, but most leading medical organizations continue to treat the nation's growing nutrition consciousness in general, and vitamin supplementation in particular, as something akin to super-stition. In such an atmosphere, the controversy over vitamin C is unlikely to subside in the near future.

Vitamin C and the Immune System

Whether or not they believe in vitamin C as a cold cure, scientists agree that ascorbic acid enhances immune respon-siveness. In a 1977 South African study, researchers in-jected college students with 1,000 milligrams of vitamin C a day for seventy-five days. Blood tests showed significant increases in levels of IgA, IgM, and C-3 complement pro-tein. Recall from chapter 3 that IgA is the body's first line of defense against upper respiratory viruses. IgM helps stimulate secretion of IgA. And C-3 complement spurs the macrophages to devour virus particles and helps trigger B-cell production of antibodies.

A 1981 study in the *Journal of Clinical Nutrition* showed that a single 1,000-milligram injection of ascorbic acid acti-vates virus-fighting neutrophils and spurs the transforma-tion of lymphocytes into virus-eating macrophages. Other recent studies show that vitamin C stimulates the produc-tion of new white blood cells and increases the release of prostaglandins, which contribute to the inflammation reac-tion.

Finally, a 1973 Scottish study shows that shortly after cold-virus infection, the level of vitamin C in white blood cells begins to fall. It drops 50 percent by the second day of symptoms, then rises slowly, returning to the preinfec-tion level after about five days. Supplementation with 200 milligrams of vitamin C has no effect on this phenomenon, but supplementation with 1,000 milligrams per day prior to cold infection and 6,000 milligrams a day while cold symp-toms are present largely prevents the vitamin C decrease and holds its level within the normal range. The authors comment that their observations "are not incompatible with the recommendations of Pauling, who suggests 1,000 to 2,000 milligrams of vitamin C every day, and 4,000 to 10,000 milligrams per day to combat cold symptoms."

Vitamin C Versus Colds: Pro and Con

Pauling's 1986 book, *How to Live Longer and Feel Better,* reviews sixteen studies that show that compared with placebo treatment, vitamin C reduces cold symptoms an average of 34 percent. In contrast, *Consumer Reports* and several other reviewers cite an equal number of studies that show no significant vitamin C effect on cold symptoms. The situation is reminiscent of the conflicting evidence for and against antihistamines. But in that case, when faced with inconsistent data, most physicians (with the notable exception of the FDA Review Panel) have endorsed antihistamines as beneficial (or at least as good placebos), while in this case, they have dismissed vitamin C as worthless. Despite medical denunciations, however, millions of people swear by vitamin C for the common cold.

Unlike antihistamines, which may cause drowsiness and imperil driving, even ascorbic acid's detractors agree that it is safe, even in doses upward of 10,000 milligrams per day. The only common side effect is diarrhea. (One report adds that it "may theoretically" trigger gout or the formation of kidney stones, but to date, these side effects have never been reported.)

Pauling's detractors never tire of citing the studies showing that vitamin C has no benefit against the common cold, but generally ignore the studies that show it to be useful. Pauling, however, does not ignore his opposition. He writes,

The principal reason for the failure of many controlled trials to show a preventive or therapeutic effect is that the amounts of vitamin C were too small . . . and because the vitamin was not taken over a long enough period of time. The proper amount is an intake just below the amount that causes a laxative effect, [which varies from] 4,000 to 15,000 mg for people in good health but grows much larger for the same people suffering from viral infection. Individual doses should be determined by people's own bowel-tolerance limits. I believe that everyone can be protected from the common cold. Catching a cold and letting it run its course is a sign that you are not taking enough vitamin C.

If you believe in vitamin C, there is no reason not to take it—even in large doses. Many studies have shown significant benefit beyond any placebo effect (itself an important healing ally). In addition, unlike many OTCs, which work by suppressing the immune system, vitamin C enhances it. Ascorbic acid is safe even in large doses, and its only significant side effect, bowel loosening, might well be a *benefit* to the millions of Americans troubled by chronic constipation.

Taking Vitamin C

At low doses (up to 250 milligrams), about 80 percent of ingested vitamin C enters the bloodstream; the rest is excreted in the urine. However, as dosage rises, the proportion absorbed falls. Only half of a 2,000-milligram dose enters the bloodstream of a healthy individual. Critics of vitamin supplementation often say that much of the money spent on vitamin C (and the other water-soluble vitamins) is literally flushed down the toilet. To ensure maximum absorption, it's better to take lower doses more frequently, except during illnesses, when one's vitamin C blood level falls and a greater proportion of higher-dose supplements is absorbed.

Top food sources of vitamin C (more than 50 milligrams per 100 grams) include broccoli, green peppers, tomato puree, brussels sprouts, citrus fruits, and cauliflower. Moderate food sources (20 to 50 milligrams per 100 grams) include: onions, melons, pineapples, tomatoes, sweet potatoes, and white cabbage.

Vitamin C deteriorates over time and with cooking. Fresh foods contain the most. Bottled fruit juices retain most of their vitamin C until opened, but once exposed to air, the vitamin content begins to deteriorate. Frozen juice concentrates also retain much of their vitamin C until mixed with water.

However, "taking" vitamin C for the common cold as Pauling advises almost always means taking supplement pills. Vitamin consumers should practice sensible supplementation and beware of misleading promotional claims. Vitamins are essential to life, but they do not "boost energy" or "control stress." Calories are the only nutrients capable of boosting energy, and although vitamins have been shown to contribute to recovery from major physical stresses, such as surgery or massive burns, they have never been shown to help alleviate everyday pressures and anxieties. Vitamins are coenzymes. They link up with the protein components of enzymes (apoenzymes) to form complete enzymes, which catalyze the chemical reactions necessary for healthy metabolism. But they do not take the place of a balanced diet.

"Natural" vitamins are no different from "synthetic." Ascorbic acid is ascorbic acid, whether it comes from rose hips, acerola cherries, or a test tube. *Natural* refers not to the vitamin itself but rather to the other ingredients: colors, flavors, fillers, binders, and coatings. Finally, there is no benefit to "chelated" or "assured absorption" vitamins. The key to vitamin C absorption is frequent low doses.

With vitamin C—and all vitamins—the more expensive brands are not necessarily the best. Most nutritionists (and Pauling himself) recommend buying the most economical brands and those with expiration dates—because vitamin potency deteriorates over time.

CHAPTER
10

Alcohol, Chicken Soup, and "...Starve a Cold"

For centuries before Linus Pauling touted bottles of vitamin C, most cold sufferers reached for bottles of something else—whiskey. Here's what a widely quoted eighteenth-century British physician prescribed, "Hang your hat on a bedpost. Get into bed and drink from a bottle of good whiskey. When two hats appear, you're on your way to recovery."

As discussed in chapter 8, alcohol is a hidden—and potentially problematic—ingredient in many OTC cold liquids. It bears repeating that alcohol is the world's most abused drug. Nonetheless, small doses may help induce the meditative state that stimulates the immune system, and larger doses have a sedative effect, which promotes rest.

Some aficionados of medicinal alcohol take it straight, but

most mix it with other ingredients to make "hot toddies."
Here are three recipes:

COGNAC TODDY
1 cup hot black tea
1 Tablespoon honey
1 Tablespoon cognac
1 teaspoon butter
¼ teaspoon cinnamon

WHISKEY TODDY
1 cup hot herb tea (see chapter 11)
4 Tablespoons Irish whiskey
2 Tablespoons lemon juice
1 Tablespoon honey

RUM TODDY
1 cup boiling water
4 Tablespoons rum
2 Tablespoons lemon juice
3 Tablespoons honey

Independent of any alcohol action, the hot water helps clear
nasal mucus, the lemon juice contains a little vitamin C, and
the honey may help soothe an irritated throat.

A similar folk remedy uses vinegar instead of alcohol.
Vinegar has no effect on cold viruses, but like its alcohol
counterparts, this toddy recipe has stood the test of time, if
not science:

WARM VINEGAR TODDY
¼ cup apple cider vinegar, warmed
¼ cup honey
Dose: 1 Tablespoon every 2 hours

Jewish Penicillin

"Soup from a fat hen" was first prescribed for the common cold eight hundred years ago by rabbi/physician Moses Maimonides. Maimonides was the court physician to Saladin, caliph of Egypt. He was so renowed that Richard the Lion-Hearted, king of England, asked him to become his personal physician. But Maimonides declined. He felt more comfortable in Cairo, where he spent much of his life writing scholarly interpretations of Jewish law.

Maimonides' cold remedy remained a hallowed, but scientifically ignored, treatment until 1978, when, on a whim, Marvin Sackner, M.D., a pulmonologist at Mount Sinai Hospital in Miami Beach, included chicken soup from a nearby delicatessen in a test of the effects of hot and cold beverages on the clearance of nasal mucus. The faster this mucus leaves the nose, the less likely it is to contribute to nasal congestion and cough. Cold water finished last, with a maximum mucus velocity of 7.8 millimeters per minute; hot water fared better, 8.4; but the chicken soup topped them both at 9.2 millimeters per minute.

Sackner wrote in the journal *Chest* that "drinking hot fluids increases nasal mucus velocity because of inhalation of heated water vapor. Hot chicken soup, either through its aroma or a mechanism related to taste, appears to possess an additional substance which increases nasal mucus velocity."

Sackner did not speculate on what this "additional substance" might be, nor did he test any other soups, so it's unclear whether Maimonides' remedy is unique or simply one of a number of equally helpful hot beverages. Sackner also cautioned that the chicken soup effect "is rather short lived, less than 30 minutes, and might not be clinically important" to cold sufferers.

But Sackner's reservations did not matter to the hordes of reporters who besieged the bewildered, suddenly famous scientist. Sackner could not understand why an experiment he considered fairly frivolous should cause such a stir. But his phone would not stop ringing, so eventually he stopped answering it. Today, a decade after his now-classic experiment, he still refuses interviews about the research that made him famous.

However, another member of the Sackner family has been more forthcoming, the scientist's mother, Goldie, also of Miami Beach. Mrs. Sackner was reportedly miffed that her son used store-bought chicken soup instead of her infinitely more therapeutic recipe. For the record:

> **GOLDIE SACKNER'S CHICKEN SOUP**
> *1 whole chicken (preferably kosher)*
> *2 carrots, chopped*
> *2 stalks celery, chopped*
> *1 onion, chopped*
> *soup greens, parsley, dill, salt and pepper to taste*

The Mount Sinai gift shop now markets its own brand of canned chicken soup (produced by Manischewitz) as "just what the doctor ordered" for colds. Sales are reportedly "brisk."

One note of caution: Canned chicken soups are usually high in salt. People on salt-restricted diets should buy low-salt brands or make their own.

". . . Starve a Cold"

The old adage, "Feed a fever, starve a cold" is difficult to take seriously because it's often heard the other way around, "Starve a fever, stuff a cold."

Authorities disagree about nutritional treatments for the common cold. Beyond encouraging hot fluids, most physicians advocate no specific food items, but do discourage deep-fried foods, which are difficult to digest. Practitioners of alternative healing arts recommend foods high in vitamin C, herb teas (see chapter 11), and avoiding meat and dairy products, which some say contribute to the secretion of excess mucus.

The meat/milk/mucus recommendation is largely based on the work of Arnold Ehret, a German naturopathic physician (1866–1922). Ehret and other nineteenth-century naturopaths rejected Pasteur's germ theory—and the vaccines and drugs developed to prevent and treat infectious diseases—in favor of rest, "water cures" at health spas, and vegetarianism to bolster the body's constitutional defenses against illness. To encourage balanced diet, a leading American naturopath, Dr. John Kellogg of Battle Creek, Michigan, invented the nation's first "health food," odd little flakes of corn. Kellogg's Corn Flakes have been popular ever since.

But by World War I, naturopathy had fallen into disrepute, a casualty of the startling successes of scientific medicine. Newly armed with the germ theory, the heirs of Louis Pasteur succeeded in preventing and curing many of the scourges that had ravaged humanity since biblical times—smallpox, typhoid, and rabies, among others.

Today, however, the major killers are no longer infectious diseases but nongerm illnesses: heart disease, stroke, and cancer, which can often be prevented or controlled using nutritional and life-style approaches similar to those advocated a century ago by naturopaths. As a result, updated naturopathy, which embraces the germ theory but largely rejects pharmaceutical drugs, is enjoying a modest comeback among those who favor nutritional approaches to health and distrust orthodox medicine's sometimes-toxic medications.

Arnold Ehret was a naturopathic maverick. He believed that the single cause of all illness was mucus and that the sticky goo should be eliminated by shunning all animal products and eating only the foods God himself provided in the Book of Genesis: fresh fruits and vegetables, nuts, herbs, and whole grains. Ehret was way off base as far as the perniciousness of mucus was concerned, but his dietary recommendations sound surprisingly contemporary. His low-fat, high-fiber diet parallels the guidelines of the American Heart Association and American Cancer Society.

For treatment of acute illnesses, Ehret recommended modified fasts of up to a month during which one subsisted solely on fruit and vegetable juices—hence, one possible derivation of ". . . starve a cold." Ehret's fasts cannot be called "starving," but they were certainly spartan.

Orthodox physicians scoff at juice fasts. They say that the nutritional key to upper respiratory infections—especially those with fever—is to drink plenty of fluids, preferably hot fluids, in order to replace those lost through excess perspiration. While endorsing hot fluids, many alternative practitioners also recommend juice fasts for a variety of illnesses, including the common cold.

11

Herbal Cold Remedies

Herbs were the original medicines, not just for the common cold but for every illness. Herbs were typically dried before they were used medicinally; the word *drug* comes from the German *droge,* which means "to dry."

Much of the world's population—maybe even a majority—still uses herbal medicines instead of pharmaceutical drugs. Many pharmaceuticals are derived from plants long valued for their healing properties. One noteworthy example is the purple-flowered foxglove. In 1775 a British physician learned from a midwife/herbalist that foxglove leaf tea helped relieve "dropsy," the heart weakness and internal fluid accumulation now known as congestive heart failure. Digitalis, the drug derived from foxglove, is still used to treat this condition.

Other examples abound. Quinine, the first drug found

effective against malaria, comes from the bark of the Peruvian cinchona tree. Raspberry leaf tea, a remedy for menstrual cramps and labor pains since the Middle Ages, was recently shown to contain substances that relax the uterus. A 1985 study in the *British Journal of Medicine* shows that feverfew (also known as bachelor's button), an ancient treatment for fever, prevents migraine headaches. Senna, a traditional herbal laxative, is the active ingredient in many OTC laxatives. And the world's oldest decongestant, ephedra, is still widely used to treat asthma and cold symptoms.

Herb Revival—and Backlash

Since the early 1970s, America has witnessed a major herb renaissance. Many people concerned about pesticides and food additives have turned away from "chemicals" and embraced what they consider to be "natural, organic" alternatives. In addition, the shortcomings of increasingly high-tech medicine have spawned what John Naisbitt's *Megatrends* calls "high-touch" reactions—the self-health and alternative health movements. Several alternative healing arts currently experiencing new or renewed popularity—chiropractic, homeopathy, naturopathy, and Chinese medicine—often prescribe herbal medicines.

Today, natural food stores and most supermarkets carry dozens of herb tea beverage blends. In addition, for the more medicinally inclined, most natural food stores also feature row upon row of large jars containing raw herbs in bulk. Nearby, collections of reference books, called herbals, purport to provide medicinal recipes for everything from insomnia to cancer. In 1985, according to the trade publication *Natural Foods Merchandiser,* herb sales at natural food stores topped $260 million, about evenly divided between blends and bulk herbs.

But as herbal popularity has grown, so has orthodox medical backlash. For the last decade, the medical journals have published a steady stream of case reports of toxic reactions. Such common herbs as chamomile, comfrey, licorice root, pennyroyal, and golden seal have allegedly caused rashes, nausea, vomiting, diarrhea, allergy attacks, miscarriage, high blood pressure, convulsions, paralysis, and even death.

"Too many people have embraced herbs uncritically," says Joe Graedon, syndicated drug columnist and co-author (with Teresa Graedon) of the *People's Pharmacy* books. "They don't trust doctors and 'drugs,' and they believe that herbs are safe, effective, and wonderful. But if herbs have beneficial effects—and there's no doubt that some do—then just like pharmaceuticals, they can also have side effects and toxic effects. Take licorice root: Many herbals recommend it for sore throat and other ailments, but it can elevate blood pressure, cause irregular heartbeat, and even contribute to heart failure."

"Because herbs are 'natural' as opposed to 'synthetic,' many people worried about carcinogens in the food supply believe that they are not hazardous," writes pharmacist David G. Spoerke, Jr., author of *Herbal Medications.* "But herbs can cause an enormous number of toxic reactions."

Herb advocates vehemently disagree. "Are herb teas dangerous? Poppycock," Norman Farnsworth, Ph.D., professor of pharmacology at the University of Illinois at Chicago, told an herbal convention in 1980. "Many of the herbs maligned in the press have been used safely for centuries, in fact, millennia."

"Do not let complicated medical works worry you to death," writes Donald Law in *The Concise Herbal Encyclopedia.* "Herbal medicine is the most reliable, most tested form of healing, proven safe over the entire history of mankind."

"The allegations against herbs are absurd," writes herb researcher Robert S. McCaleb in the trade journal *Health Foods Retailing.* "Herbs have been used as beverages and medicines since before recorded history. A few problems have surfaced. But the press has sensationalized them badly. Considering the millions of people who consume herb teas daily, there have really been very few problems."

Dosage Control

The truth about herb safety lies somewhere between the unqualified endorsements in some herbals and the dire warnings in the medical journals. With good information, consumers *can* use herbs safely to treat many illnesses, including the common cold.

The crux of the matter is dose control. The FDA requires OTC pharmaceutical packaging to specify precisely how much active ingredient each tablet contains, how often the drug may be taken, and warnings about possible side effects, with additional warnings for those at special risk, for example, pregnant women. But medicinal herbs sold in bulk typically lack sufficient cautionary labeling and dosage-control information.

Suppose, for example, an herbal recommends one ounce of herb in a pint of boiled water. Without sophisticated laboratory equipment, it's impossible to know how much active ingredient the tea contains and how many cups of the brew might cause problems. Many factors affect an herb's potency: genetics, farming methods, maturity at harvest, time in storage, and steeping time. Consider coffee: Depending on the variety, roast, freshness, and brewing method, a tablespoon of coffee beans can produce a beverage with a tremendous range of caffeine content.

"Many people believe that if a little of something is good, then more must be better," Spoerke says. "That's naive. Most toxic reactions to herbs do not involve people who drink a few cups a day of the beverage blends. They involve people who self-medicate with literally *gallons* of tea brewed from pharmacologically active herbs. It's amazing how many people use herbs with no understanding of dose control—and wind up regretting it."

Commercial beverage blends rarely cause problems, even for heavy users. However, large amounts of two common herbs—chamomile and licorice root—might possibly cause problems (see "Herbal Teas for Cold Symptoms," below). The herbs most likely to cause adverse reactions are the ones sold in bulk.

Natural food stores, where most bulk herbs are sold, handle herb safety issues differently. A 1984 survey by *Natural Foods Merchandiser* showed that 61 percent relied on verbal warnings from sales staff; 55 percent declined to carry potentially toxic herbs; 29 percent attached cautionary labels to certain jars; 14 percent took no precautions; and 10 percent placed warnings on the walls near their herb sections. (Many stores took more than one type of precaution.) In general, the larger the store, the fewer the precautions.

The precautions taken by natural food stores depend to a large extent on well-informed salespeople. Presumably, the staff who provide the warnings have read herbals. But there's the rub. Few herbals take safety issues seriously enough.

Consumers interested in herbal medicine should not rely on checkout-counter advice. They should take responsibility for their use of medicinal herbs. Several good herbals are recommended in resources.

FDA-Approved Herbs for Colds

The herbs used to treat upper respiratory infections should not be considered "cures." Some may stimulate immune responsiveness, but like the OTCs, they provide mostly symptomatic relief.

Herbal remedies for the common cold may be divided into three groups—those FDA-approved as "safe and effective," those approved as "safe," and those not discussed by the FDA OTC Review Panel. Recall from chapter 8 that *safe and effective* means that the FDA Review Panel found consistent evidence of efficacy and safety at recommended doses. *Safe* means that the remedy has been widely used for many years without significant reports of adverse effects, but may or may not be effective. Finally, the herbs not discussed by the FDA have *not* been prohibited by the federal agency. They have simply been ignored. Although many have been used to treat cold symptoms for centuries, they are not commonly used in OTC cold formulas, so the FDA Review Panel saw no reason to rule on them.

The following herbs are FDA-approved as safe and effective:

• *Camphor oil. Approved as a cough suppressant.* The oil of the camphor tree is safe and effective when inhaled or used in ointments. The FDA permits up to 5.3 percent camphor oil in OTC cold remedies. However, camphor should not be ingested; it is highly toxic even at low doses.

• *Ephedra. Approved as a decongestant.* Also known as Mormon tea, desert tea, and mahuang (see chapter 12), its active ingredient is ephedrine. The FDA allows up to 1 percent ephedrine in OTC cold remedies. Like pseudoephedrine, ephedra increases blood pressure and should not be used by those with diabetes, heart disease, high blood pressure, or a history of stroke. It may also cause insomnia. (For tea, see next section.)

• *Eucalyptus/eucalyptus oil/eucalyptol. Approved as a cough suppressant.* The aromatic eucalyptus is also known as the Australian fever tree, because its oil was once used to treat malaria. The FDA permits up to 1.3 percent eucalyptol in OTC cold remedies. (For tea, see next section.)

• *Peppermint/peppermint oil/menthol. Approved as a cough suppressant.* Mint leaves have been used since ancient times to treat colds, cough, and indigestion. A vestige of this herb's digestive use survives today in the after-dinner mint. The FDA allows up to 2.8 percent peppermint in OTC cold remedies. Peppermint oil, also known as menthol, is used in lozenges, inhalants, ointments, and salves. In doses greater than 5,000 milligrams, peppermint oil may cause drowsiness and vomiting. (For tea, see next section.)

The following herbs are FDA-approved as safe:

• *Belladonna. Approved as an anticholinergic drying agent.* Its common name is "deadly nightshade," and *deadly* is no joke. Even small amounts of this herb may cause delirium, hallucinations, and death. Minute amounts are incorporated into some OTC cold remedies, but the plant material should *never* be ingested.

• *Cedar leaf oil. Approved as a topical decongestant.* This aromatic oil smells like turpentine and is approved for use in salves and ointments. Cedar leaf oil should not be ingested. Thujone, a component of the oil, stimulates uterine contractions, possibly causing miscarriage, and at high doses it causes convulsion, coma, and death.

• *Horehound. Approved as a cough suppressant.* A popular folk remedy for respiratory complaints, this member of the mint family has been used for centuries to treat coughs and sore throats. The FDA has set no dosage limits for the OTC lozenges and syrups that include it. (For tea, see next section.)

• *Peppermint/camphor/eucalyptus. Approved as decongestants and expectorants.* See above. (For teas, see next section.)

• *Slippery elm bark. Approved as a cough suppressant.* Indians, slaves, and pioneers used it to treat fever, colds, cough, and sore throat. No toxic ingestions have ever been reported, but skin rash is possible. (For tea, see next section.)

• *Thyme oil/thymol. Approved as a topical cough suppressant and decongestant.* The ancient Greeks used thyme to treat fever, cough, bronchitis, and asthma. The FDA has set no dosage limits for ointments and salves containing thymol, but the potent oil should not be ingested. As little as .2 milliliters may cause nausea and vomiting. However, the less potent leaves may be brewed into tea, (see next section).

Most herb tea companies produce "beverages" and are prohibited from mentioning that some of their ingredients might have pharmacological effects. However, two herb companies—Traditional Medicinals of Rohnert Park, California, and McZand Herbal, Inc., of Santa Monica, California—are FDA-licensed *drug* companies. They are free to make medicinal claims for their dose-controlled herbal cold remedies. Dosage information appears on product packaging. They also provide warnings about overdose and risks to pregnant women, children, and those with chronic illnesses. The active ingredients in their cold formulas are ephedra, peppermint, and slippery elm. Other herbs are added for flavor (see resources).

Among FDA-approved herbal cold remedies, ephedra, like its cousin psuedoephedrine, suppresses capillary dilation in the nasopharynx and works against the immune system's cold-healing efforts. The immune system effects of most other herbal cold remedies remain unclear. Some may enhance immune response. Others may suppress it. All may stimulate the self-healing placebo effect.

Herb Teas for Cold Symptoms

Down through the ages, dozens of other herbs have been used to treat cold symptoms. Different herbals recommend different herbs, in widely differing amounts, prepared differently, with different warnings (if any) about safe dose limits and the possible effects of overdose. This often frustrates those who would like to use herbal cold remedies confidently and safely. It also bolsters the view of herb critics who charge that herbals often recommend "any amount of any herb any time for any illness."

Nonetheless, what follows is a composite list of herbs mentioned as cold remedies by the herbals cited in resources. These herbals inspire greater confidence than most because they rely on more than folklore. They cite scientific research concerning therapeutic and adverse effects and attempt to specify dosage limits.

Unfortunately, these references also disagree. In cases where they disagree about dosage, I present the most conservative recommendation. (All dosage information applies to *adults only.* For children's doses, see chapter 16.) Where they disagree about effectiveness, I note the disagreement. Where they disagree about possible adverse effects, I take the conservative position, and mention all potential side effects—but bear in mind that unless otherwise specified, serious adverse reactions appear only at enormous doses. Finally, in cases where recent research has shown an herb to contain even the smallest trace of a carcinogen, mutagen (mutation-causing substance), or other toxic chemical, that information is noted.

Although I advocate conservatism in the use of medicinal herbs (and all drugs), at the same time this book aims to empower readers with a realistic view of herb safety. After all, several people die each year from overdoses of aspirin, but realistically, aspirin is quite valuable, and consumers need not fear serious problems from occasional use—as long as they are aware of the caveats discussed in chapter 8. Given all the conflicting information about herb safety, we are fortunate that James A. Duke, Ph.D., chief of the U.S. Department of Agriculture's Medicinal Plant Laboratory for twenty-five years, has published what in my opinion is the best herbal, the encyclopedic *CRC Handbook of Medici-*

nal Herbs (see resources). After analyzing all reports of toxic reactions, he developed the following ranking system:

0   *Very dangerous. Duke would not ingest any.*

1   *More hazardous than coffee. Duke would limit consumption to one cup a day while symptoms persist.*

2   *About as hazardous as coffee. Duke would limit consumption to two cups a day while symptoms persist.*

3   *Safer than coffee. Duke wouldn't hesitate to drink three cups a day for symptoms.*

X   *Essentially safe. No safety questions have been raised, but some individuals might be allergic.*

After presenting the potential adverse effects discussed in the other herbals, each herb discussed below is given a bottom-line "Duke ranking."

Many medicinal herbs taste quite bitter. It often helps to add lemon or honey or mix them with an herbal beverage blend.

• *Angelica. Recommended for colds and cough.* Mix 1 teaspoon of the root in 1 pint of boiled water, then steep for 30 minutes. Cool in a closed container. Take 1 tablespoon at a time, up to 1 cup a day. Or mix ½ ounce of leaves in 1 pint of boiled water and steep for 5 to 20 minutes (the longer, the stronger). Take up to 2 cups a day. Angelica should not be used by pregnant women. It promotes menstruation and at high doses can induce abortion and cause poisoning. Sources disagree about the advisability of taking angelica internally, because recent research shows that it contains mutagens. Duke ranking: 2.

• *Basil. Recommended for colds and flu.* Mix 1 ounce with 1 pint of boiled water and steep for 5 to 20 minutes. Little has been written about the medicinal use or potential toxicity of this common kitchen herb. Duke ranking: 2.

• *Cayenne. Recommended for colds and flu.* Mix ¼ to 1 teaspoon per cup of boiled water. Take 1 or 2 cups per day. This hot red pepper produces an immediate sensation of heat and is usually recommended as a digestive stimulant. Sources disagree about its use for colds and flu. Large doses may cause diarrhea, nausea, and vomiting. Those with gastrointestinal ulcers, colitis, or other bowel conditions should not use cayenne. Duke ranking: 2.

• *Chamomile. Recommended for colds and flu.* Mix ½ to 1 ounce per pint of boiled water; steep for 10 minutes. Chamomile is one of the most widely used beverage and medicinal herbs. Included in many packaged blends, it is also recommended for its calming, sleep-inducing, and general "tonic" effects. Sources dispute its effectiveness against colds. Chamomile is generally considered nontoxic even at high doses, but there have been some reports of allergic reactions in those sensitive to ragweed. Duke ranking: 3.

• *Coltsfoot. Recommended for cough.* Mix 1 ounce per pint of boiled water. Take 1 or 2 cups per day. Hippocrates prescribed coltsfoot for cough, and this herb's Latin name, *Tussilago* is derived from *tussis,* which means "cough." No poisonings have ever been reported, but sources disagree about the advisability of taking coltsfoot internally—recent research has shown it to contain a carcinogen, senkirkine. Large doses have caused liver tumors in laboratory animals. Duke ranking: 2.

• *Comfrey. Recommended for cough.* Soak 2 ounces in 1 quart of water overnight; simmer for 30 minutes, then strain. Add 6 ounces of honey. Take 2 tablespoons 3 or 4 times a day. Comfrey is often regarded as an herbal panacea. One herbal says it "has a healing effect on every organ in the body." Perhaps, but recent research shows that this herb contains several carcinogens. The safety of comfrey is hotly debated in herbal circles. Duke ranking: 2.

• *Elder flowers. Recommended for colds, flu, and fever.* Mix 1 ounce of herb per pint of boiled water; steep for 5 to 20 minutes. Take 1 or 2 cups a day. A laxative effect is possible. Overdose produces nausea and vomiting. Duke ranking: 1.

• *Ephedra. Recommended for colds, flu, cough, and congestion.* An FDA-approved treatment for congestion—see previous section. For tea, mix ½ ounce per pint of boiled water, and steep for 5 to 20 minutes. Take 1 to 2 cups per day. Ephedra elevates blood pressure and should not be used by those with diabetes, heart disease, high blood pressure, or a history of stroke. It may also cause insomnia. Duke ranking: 1.

• *Eucalyptus. Recommended for cough and congestion.* An FDA-approved cough suppressant—see previous section. For tea, use 1 teaspoon of crushed leaves per pint of boiled water, and steep for 5 to 20 minutes. Take up to 2 cups per day. Duke ranking: 2.

• *Garlic. Recommended for colds and flu.* To prepare garlic oil, place 8 ounces of peeled, minced cloves in a jar. Add enough olive oil to cover it and allow to stand for 3 days, shaking a few times a day. Strain, discard the cloves, and store the oil in a cool place. Take 1 teaspoon of garlic oil per hour while symptoms persist. Garlic has been used medicinally since ancient times. Several cloves were found in King Tut's tomb. During the Middle Ages (and until quite recently in some cultures), garlic cloves were worn around the neck, and braids and wreaths were hung in homes, to prevent illness and possession by evil spirits. Garlic contains an amino acid derivative, alliin. When crushed or minced, the enzyme allinase is released, which converts the alliin to allicin. Allicin is an antibiotic equivalent to 1 percent penicillin. Garlic also thins the blood and prevents clotting, which may help control high blood pressure and prevent heart attack. Garlic has no known antiviral activity, and herbals dispute its effectiveness, but it has been used to treat colds for centuries. Garlic is nontoxic in adults, but there have been a few reports of reactions to extraordinarily large doses in children. Duke ranking: X.

• *Ginger. Recommended for colds and flu.* Mix 1 ounce of grated root per pint of boiled water. Take up to 2 cups a day. No reports of toxicity. Duke ranking: X.

• *Horehound. Recommended for cough and congestion.* An FDA-approved cough suppressant—see previous section. For tea, mix 1 teaspoon of leaves and/or flowers per pint of boiled water. When cool, take 1 tablespoon every few hours (very bitter). Large doses may cause diarrhea and nausea. Duke ranking: X.

• *Hyssop. Recommended for colds, flu, cough, congestion, and fever.* Mix 1 ounce of herb per pint of boiled water. The volatile oil, similar to angelica, helps soothe the respiratory tract. No reports of toxicity. Duke ranking: X.

• *Lemon balm. Recommended for colds, flu, fever.* Mix 2 teaspoons per cup of boiled water, then steep for 5 minutes. Take 1 tablespoon every few hours. Sources disagree about its effectiveness. No reports of toxicity. Duke ranking: X.

• *Licorice. Recommended for sore throat, colds, flu.* Add a pinch of crushed or powdered root to beverage teas. Licorice contains glycyrrhizin, chemically similar to the adrenal hormone aldosterone. Excessive amounts may produce pseudoaldosteronism: headache, lethargy, sodium and water retention, elevated blood pressure, and at high doses, possibly heart failure. Those with diabetes, high blood pressure, heart disease or a history of stroke should not use licorice. Duke ranking: 1.

• *Onion. Recommended for colds and flu.* At the first sign of a cold or flu, chew fresh onion. Related to garlic, similar claims have been made for it throughout history. Sources disagree on its effectiveness against colds. No reports of toxicity. Duke ranking: X.

• *Peppermint. Recommended for colds, flu, cough, and congestion.* An FDA-approved cough suppressant, expectorant, and decongestant. For tea, mix ½ ounce of leaves per pint of boiled water and steep for 5 to 20 minutes. No limit on adult consumption, but peppermint tea is not recommended for infants and young children because its pungent fragrance may trigger choking (see chapter 16). Duke ranking: X.

• *Pleurisy root. Recommended for cough.* Boil ½ teaspoon of powdered root in 1 pint of water for 30 minutes. Cool in a closed container. Take 1 tablespoon every few hours, up to 1 cup per day. Large doses produce weakness, loss of appetite, gastrointestinal upsets, diarrhea, and possibly even death from respiratory paralysis. Duke ranking: 1.

• *Propolis. Recommended for colds and flu.* Propolis is not really an herb, but "bee glue," pine resin used by bees to fill cracks in their hives. Studies show that it has mild antibacterial and fungicidal properties and that it accelerates tissue regeneration. But propolis has not been shown effective against cold viruses. Available as a powder or in capsules or lozenges. No reports of toxicity. Duke ranking: none.

• *Sage. Recommended for colds and flu.* Mix ¼ ounce per pint of boiled water, then steep for 10 minutes. Take no more than 3 cups a day for 10 days. Sage contains thujones, which cause convulsions in large doses. Duke ranking: 3.

• *Sarsparilla. Recommended for colds, cough, fever.* Boil ½ teaspoon of root in 1 pint of water for 30 minutes. Cool in a closed container. Take 1 tablespoon every few hours, up to 2 cups a day. Sources disagree on its effectiveness against cold symptoms. Sarsparilla has diuretic and laxative properties at large doses. No reports of toxicity. Duke ranking: 2.

• *Slippery elm bark. Recommended for colds, flu, cough, fever, and sore throat.* An FDA-approved cough suppressant—see previous section. For tea, mix 1 teaspoon of bark per pint of water. Boil for 30 minutes, then cool. Take 1 tablespoon every few hours, up to 2 cups per day. No toxic ingestions have been reported, but skin rash is possible. Duke ranking: 2.

• *Spearmint. Recommended for colds, flu, and cough.* Mix ½ ounce per pint of boiled water and steep for 5 to 20 minutes. Very similar to peppermint. No reports of toxicity in adults, but the pungent aroma may trigger choking in infants and young children, and children may become ill after ingesting as little as 5 milligrams of the oil. Duke ranking: X.

• *Thyme. Recommended for fever, cough, and congestion.* Thyme oil is FDA-approved as a topical cough suppressant and decongestant—see previous section. For tea, mix ½ ounce per pint of boiled water; steep for 5 to 20 minutes. Take 1 or 2 cups a day for symptoms. Duke ranking: 2.

• *Yarrow. Recommended for colds, flu.* Mix ½ ounce per pint of boiled water, steep for 5 to 20 minutes. Take 2 or 3 cups per day. Sources disagree about effectiveness. A relative of chamomile, generally nontoxic, but may cause allergic reactions in those sensitive to ragweed. Duke ranking: 3.

RESOURCES

Traditional Medicinals. 215 Classic Court, Rohnert Park, Calif. 94928. Produces the following FDA-approved OTC cold products: Breathe Easy for nasal and bronchial congestion; active ingredient: ephedra. Gypsy Cold Care for colds: peppermint. Throat Coat for sore throat: licorice root. Available at natural food stores, some pharmacies and supermarkets, and from the *Self-Care Catalog,* 11 Chapel St., Augusta, Me. 04330; (207) 622-5949

. . .

McZand Herbals, Inc. P.O. Box 5312, Santa Monica, Calif. 90405. Produces the following FDA-approved OTC cold products: HerbaLozenge for sore throat and cough; active ingredient: peppermint. Decongest Herbal for nasal congestion: ephedra.

The CRC Handbook of Medicinal Herbs by James A. Duke, Ph.D. 1985, $195.00 from CRC Press, 2000 Corporate Boulevard, N.W., Boca Raton, Fla. 33431. The definitive herbal. Very expensive but worth it for the herb enthusiast who wants an encyclopedic resource.

The Way of Herbs by Michael Tierra, C.A., N.D. 1983, $4.95 from Washington Square Press, 1230 Avenue of the Americas, New York, N.Y. 10020. More folklore than science, but comprehensive, with a good chapter on herb safety.

Herbal Medications by David Spoerke, Jr., M.S. 1980, $5.95 from Woodbridge Press, P.O. Box 6189, Santa Barbara, Calif. 93111. Brief scientific summaries of herbal safety. Very conservative.

The Honest Herbal by Varro Tyler, Ph.D. 1983, $14.50 from G. F. Stickley Co., 210 West Washington Square, Philadelphia, Pa. 19106. Scientific discussions of medicinal herbs. Very conservative.

C H A P T E R
12

Traditional Chinese Cold Cures

"Of all the experiences I have had in America," writes Hong Liu, a scholar from a family of traditional Chinese physicians, who spent 1984 in the United States preparing to study medicine, "nothing has surprised me more than Americans' belief that there is no cure for the common cold. My wonderment at this led me to consult several medical books, which only increased my bewilderment. I found that the commonly recommended treatments are considered 'largely palliative,' and not curative. As one who has always been cured of colds whenever afflicted in my native land, I make the outlandish claim that the common cold and flu can be cured. Chinese medicine cures what Western medicine is powerless against." Hong Liu's attitude is typical of Chinese medical authorities, who view the orthodox West-

ern approach—symptomatic relief until the body heals itself—with amused condescension.

To most Americans, "traditional Chinese medicine"
means acupuncture, the ancient art of inserting needles into
the skin at therapeutic points along energy pathways
("meridians"). In the Chinese view, the needles release
blocked vital energy, or "ch'i." Once unblocked, ch'i flows
properly, relieving pain, curing illness, and restoring mind/
body harmony. But acupuncture is only part of traditional
Chinese medicine. Herbology is actually more important,
and both are used to treat colds.

Acupressure Massage

Acupuncture was an exotic curiosity in the United States
until 1971, when Richard Nixon became the first president
to visit the People's Republic. During his visit, network
television broadcast astonishing footage of a woman undergoing abdominal surgery while fully conscious—her only
anesthesia, a few acupuncture needles in her ear lobes and
feet. *New York Times* columnist James Reston witnessed
acupuncture anesthesia firsthand and later used it successfully to help control his own pain following appendectomy.
Reston's widely publicized experience stimulated tremendous interest in the ancient healing art.

Legend has it that acupuncture developed as a result of
warfare. Ancient Chinese warriors noticed that superficial
spear and arrow wounds in certain places seemed to relieve
pain and cure illness. Centuries of literally hit-and-miss ob-
servation located the meridians, which correspond roughly
to the major nerve lines, and catalogued the energy points
along them. Recent research suggests that acupuncture al-
leviates pain by releasing endorphins, the body's own opi-
atelike painkillers. Today, there are twenty-five

acupuncture schools throughout the United States and about five thousand practicing acupuncturists.

Acupuncturists claim good success treating early-stage upper respiratory infections; however, most practice in California, eliminating this option for much of the country. Besides, from a self-care perspective, why spend the time and money on an office visit when a do-it-yourself offshoot of acupuncture may work just as well? The offshoot, acupressure, uses the same energy points but substitutes deep finger massage for acupuncture's needles.

There are just two steps to using acupressure: finding the right point and applying the proper pressure. To find the precise location of any point, press the tip of the index finger—not the pad—into the approximate location as indicated in the descriptions below. The point announces itself with a sharp twinge of sensitivity. If you don't feel the twinge, you haven't found the point. Keep probing.

Once you've found the point, apply moderate pressure by wiggling your fingertip into it. The pressure may hurt a bit, but it does no harm. Acupressurists believe that the moment of discomfort helps unblock the ch'i trapped at the point. Apply pressure for about thirty seconds, then switch to the same point on the opposite side of the body.

Although acupressure is safe and effective, it should not be used within a half hour of eating or drinking alcohol; or if the desired point lies beneath a scar, wart, mole, varicose vein or other skin blemish; or by pregnant women—it may stimulate premature labor.

All the points used to treat upper respiratory symptoms are discussed in the books listed in resources, but here are six of the most widely recommended:

• *Ta-Chui. Recommended for colds, fever, chest congestion, and bronchitis.* At the base of the neck, where the lowest neck (cervical) vertebra meets the highest upper chest (thoracic) vertebra.

- *Chih-Tse. Recommended for sore throat and cough.* On the elbow crease, one thumb-width out from the center of the arm (away from the body).
- *Ho-Ku. Recommended for headache and sore throat.* On the hand, in the center of the fleshy triangle formed between the thumb and index finger.
- *Chu-Chih. Recommended for colds and fever.* On the outside of the arm, at the end of the elbow crease when the arm is bent.
- *Ying-Hsiang. Recommended for runny nose.* Half a thumb-width away from the base of the nostril.
- *Feng-Chih. Recommended for colds.* On the back of the neck, in the hollow created by the union of the head and neck, on a line with the bottom of the ear lobe.

After applying pressure for thirty seconds to both sides of the body, rest for a few minutes, then repeat.

Chinese Herbology

Chinese herbal medicine dates back to about 250 B.C., when the book *Shan Ching* ("The Classic on the Mountain") first discussed medicinal herbs, including the decongestant mahuang (ephedra). But it took another five hundred years for China's first great herbal to appear. *Pen Tsao Ching* ("The Classic of Herbs") was written about A.D. 250 by Shen Nung, a sage who tested dozens of medicinal herbs on himself and recorded their benefits and side effects. Legend has it that he was fatally poisoned by a toxic herb. Later herbalists elaborated upon Shen Nung's work, notably Tao Hung Ching, who discussed 365 herbs in a commentary that appeared around A.D. 500.

For another one thousand years, herbalists added their experiences to Chinese herbal lore, resulting in hundreds of contradictory commentaries. In the sixteenth century, the naturalist Li Shih Chen attempted to make sense of the conflicting claims in the many herbals of his day. In 1590, Li released his landmark herbal, *Pen Tsao Kang Mu* ("The Catalog of Medicinal Herbs"), which lists more than fifteen hundred medicinal herbs and about eighteen thousand therapeutic and tonic recipes. Since Li's time, Chinese herbalists have tried to simplify their art. Today, traditional Chinese physicians use about five hundred herbs, of which two hundred are commonly prescribed.

Chinese medicine is completely different from Western medicine. No summary here could explain it. Those interested should read Ted J. Kaptchuk's excellent *The Web That Has No Weaver,* listed in resources.

Very briefly, traditional Chinese medicine does not recognize the germ theory of illness. Instead, diseases are grouped into three broad categories: physical injuries, sickness due to outward causes (for example, changes in the weather), and sickness due to inward causes (for example, changes in mood). Disease is largely conceived in terms of imbalances among the body's energy, organ, constitutional, and emotional systems. As a result, the goal of Chinese medicine is not to kill pathogens but rather to restore harmony and balance by adjusting the person's ch'i, constitution, and other factors.

The Chinese consider everyone's constitution—and virtually everything in the natural world—as unique combinations of two primary forces, *yin* and *yang,* which are both opposite and complementary. Yin is feminine, cold, pale, wet, weak, inhibited, and inwardly focused. Yin foods include fruits and vegetables. Yin herbs include chamomile, ephedra, elder, and comfrey. Yang is masculine, hot, flushed, dry, energetic, excited, and outwardly focused. Yang foods include meats, poultry, and fish. Yang herbs include ginseng, dandelion, ginger, and rhubarb.

Diseases are classified according to the "Eight Principles": Yin or Yang, Interior or Exterior, Hot or Cold, and Deficiency or Excess. To bring the Eight Principles back into healthy balance, Chinese physicians create herbal formulas grouped according to four properties, six tastes, and ten effects. The four properties include: cold, cool, warm, and hot. The six tastes: sour, bitter, sweet, salty, spicy, and tasteless. The ten effects: tonic, purgative, sedative, decongestant, diuretic, laxative, drying, moistening, sweat-releasing, and ch'i-retaining.

Diseases are also linked to one of the five major organs—heart, lung, spleen, liver, and kidney—and relate to one or more of about two dozen different kinds of pulses. The character of one's pulse is as fundamental to Chinese medicine as blood pressure is to its Western counterpart. Chinese physicians often spend several minutes feeling a patient's pulse.

No "Colds" and "Flu"

The terms *common cold* and *flu* did not exist in the Chinese vocabulary until the introduction of Western, germ-theory medicine at the turn of the century. Today, many traditional Chinese physicians still do not use these terms, though they are widely used in everyday life.

Chinese physicians classify colds and flu as sicknesses due to outward causes—wind, cold, and damp weather. Within this broad category, upper respiratory infections are associated with the lung and classified among the diseases having fever as a symptom. From the traditional Chinese perspective, fever is caused by the struggle between the person's disease resistance and the imbalances caused by the disease process. The Chinese view fever as a reassuring sign of a strong individual with good resistance. Colds and flu are further subdivided by their other symptoms—headache, runny nose, nasal congestion, cough, sneezing, aching neck, and abhorrence of cold.

Chinese medicine recognizes two major types of upper respiratory infection, Wind Cold (a yin condition) and

Wind Heat (yang). The symptoms of a Wind Cold include chills, fever, sneezing, runny nose with white mucus, and a thin white coating on the tongue. Wind Heat symptoms include sore throat, dry mouth, few or no chills, yellow nasal mucus, and a yellow coating on the tongue. Although it's difficult to make comparisons to Western classifications, Wind Cold suggests flu, whereas Wind Heat suggests the common cold.

Like Western drug companies, the Chinese have developed over-the-counter cold medicines that are available all over China and Taiwan, as well as in the United States (see resources). They come in pills, capsules, and packets used to make tea.

The herbs in Chinese cold formulas with translatable English names include: licorice, ginger, cinnamon, honeysuckle, mint, burdock, ephedra, apricot seed, and forsythia flower. However, quite a few Chinese medicinal herbs have no English translations and are identified by either their Latin or their Chinese names: Lophatherum, Schizonepeta, Bupleurum, Cnidium, and Tang-kuei, among others.

None of the preformulated traditional Chinese cold cures listed in resources come with any warnings about those who should avoid them. All the herb safety issues raised in chapter 11 also apply to Chinese herbs. Pregnant women should not use these medicines (see chapter 15). Chinese ephedra (mahuang) is much stronger than its Western relative, and its side effects are more pronounced. Many Chinese herbs have not been studied by Western scientists, so their side effects, if any, remain unclear. A few Chinese cold formulas now also contain some Western drugs. Those unfamiliar with Chinese OTCs should use them conservatively. If you have any significant health problems, consult a Chinese physician before using these cold remedies, or don't use them.

For those interested in brewing their own Chinese cold medicines, here are two recipes:

EPHEDRA HERB TEA (MAHUANG TANG)
1 tablespoon ephedra
1 tablespoon apricot seed
2 teaspoons cinnamon
¾ teaspoon ground licorice root

Simmer for one hour in a pint of boiled water in a nonmetallic pot. Take 1 cup a day. This formula is recommended for those whose upper respiratory infections involve congestion and aching joints without perspiration. Duke rates licorice and American (weaker) ephedra: 1; cinnamon: 2; and does not mention apricot seed.

CINNAMON/GINGER HERB TEA (KUEI CHIH TANG)
2 teaspoons cinnamon
2 teaspoons ginger
2 teaspoons peony alba
2 teaspoons jujube (Chinese date)
1 teaspoon ground licorice root

Simmer for 1 hour in a pint of boiled water in a nonmetallic pot. Take 1 cup a day. This formula is recommended for those whose upper respiratory infections involve headache, chills, perspiration, and digestive upset, for example, diarrhea. Duke rates licorice: 1; cinnamon: 2; ginger: X; and does not mention peony or jujube.

RESOURCES

The Natural Healer's Acupressure Handbook by Michael Blate, 1983, $14.50 postpaid from Falkynor Books, P.O. Box 8060, Hollywood, Fla. 33084; (305) 791-1562. A quick guide to 116 of the most frequently used points.

The Complete Book of Acupuncture by Stephen T. Chang, 1976, $8.95 from Celestial Arts, P.O. Box 7327, Berkeley, Calif.

94707. A comprehensive discussion of acupuncture, applicable to acupressure as well.

The Web That Has No Weaver: Understanding Chinese Medicine by Ted J. Kaptchuk, 1983, $11.95 from Congdon and Weed, 298 Fifth Avenue, New York, N.Y. 10001; or $13.95 postpaid from China Books, 2929-24th Street, San Francisco, Calif. 94110; (415) 282-2994. The best introduction to traditional Chinese medicine.

Oriental Healing Arts Institute (OHAI), a nonprofit educational organization founded in 1976 by Brion Corporation (see below), publishes dozens of books and bulletins on Chinese medicine. Write for a free catalog: OHAI, 1945 Palo Verde Avenue, Suite 208, Long Beach, Calif. 90815; (213) 431-3544.

Cold Medicines from the People's Republic of China. Ganmao Tuire Chongji—half-ounce plastic packets filled with brown granules of forsythia and other herbs; mix with boiled water to make tea, six packets, $6.00. Yin Chiao—pale green pills containing: honeysuckle, forsythia, licorice, mint, burdock, antelope horn, Lophatherum, Schizonepeta, and two Western drugs, acetaminophen and chlorpheniramine; 120 pills $6.00. Add $2 for postage and handling. From Min An Health Center, 1144 Pacific Street, San Francisco, Calif. 94133; (415) 771-4040.

Cold Medicines from Taiwan. Yin Chiao #440—honeysuckle, forsythia, and other herbs; 100 capsules, $9.80. Yin Chiao #744—Schizonepeta, forsythia, and other herbs; 100 capsules, $18.40. M-H Combination #528—mahuang ephedra, cinnamon, licorice, and apricot seed; 100 capsules $9.80. Cinnamon Combination #212—cinnamon, ginger, peony, licorice, and Chinese date; 100 capsules, $9.50. Add $3 for postage and handling. From Brion Corporation, 12020-B Centralia Road, Hawaiian Gardens, Calif. 90716; (213) 924-8875. Brion also publishes an extensive catalog of traditional Chinese herbal medicines, available free from the address above.

13

Homeopathic Cold Cures

Orthodox and herbal medicine view cold symptoms as the problem and endeavor to suppress them until the body heals itself—even if it means working against the immune system's best efforts to fight the infection. Homeopathy, on the other hand, views symptoms as expressions of the body's defenses and strives to enhance, rather than suppress, the immune system's illness-fighting efforts. In this context, homeopaths say that their cold medicines are cures.

Homeopathy is a two hundred-year-old healing art developed by Samuel Hahnemann (1755–1843), a German physician who became disillusioned with the "heroic medicine" of his day because the heroism was entirely on the part of the patient. In the late eighteenth century, physicians routinely treated the sick with bloodletting, leeches, toxic mercury-based laxatives, and nonantiseptic surgery, which Hahnemann decided (correctly) did more harm than good. Rather than cause additional suffering, he quit practicing medicine and worked instead as a medical writer and translator.

Hahnemann became fascinated by Hippocrates' accounts of treatment with "similars," the idea that substances that cause certain symptoms in healthy people cure the illnesses that cause the same symptoms. Since Hippocrates, the use of similars had remained an undercurrent in European medicine, with various physicians throughout history keeping the idea quietly alive. Hahnemann decided to test some similars on himself.

He took quinine, used to treat malaria, and found that he temporarily developed the symptoms of the disease. He tried other similars, catalogued the symptoms they caused, and began prescribing them to his family and friends for illnesses involving those symptoms. Hahnemann obtained what he considered impressive results and returned to medicine—but this time he based his practice on applications of his Law of Similars. Hahnemann's therapeutics were less drastic and less likely to harm than the often-toxic medicines prescribed by his contemporaries. Hahnemann treated many people successfully, and as word spread, he and other physicians who adopted his method developed a substantial following throughout Europe.

Early nineteenth-century German immigrants brought homeopathy to the United States. In 1833 Dr. Constantine Hering founded the nation's first homeopathic medical school in Allentown, Pennsylvania. By 1900, there were twenty-two schools, and at the time, an estimated 25 percent of U.S. physicians—some fourteen thousand practitioners—used homeopathic medicines in their practices.

Throughout the mid- and late-nineteenth century, homeopathy was quite popular in this country. Such noted

Americans as Mark Twain, Daniel Webster, Henry Wadsworth Longfellow, William James, and John D. Rockefeller preferred homeopathy to conventional "allopathic" medicine. Homeopaths pioneered the use of nitroglycerine to treat angina and ergot derivatives to treat migraine headaches—both of which are still used today. In fact, the founding of the American Medical Association (AMA) in 1846 was, in part, an attempt to compete with the rival American Institute of Homeopathy, founded two years earlier.

But with the advent of the germ theory and the rise of contemporary medicine, homeopathy was attacked as unscientific by the increasingly influential AMA, which expelled members who combined the two approaches. In 1904 the AMA established its Council on Medical Education, which published reports attacking homeopathy and other healing arts the organization considered unsound. In 1910, the Council commissioned Abraham Flexner, of the Carnegie Endowment (a key source of medical-school funding) to evaluate the nation's medical-education programs. Flexner's influential report savaged both homeopathic medicine and its schools. In short order, state medical-licensing boards stopped certifying homeopaths. Funding for homeopathic education dried up. By 1918, only six schools remained. The last one closed in 1940.

Nonetheless, homeopathy remained popular in Europe, South America, and India, which has 100,000 homeopaths, about one-quarter of whom are also M.D.'s. The physician to the British royal family is a homeopath, and in a 1985 survey by *The Times* of London, 48 percent of British general practitioners said they recommended homeopathic remedies to some of their patients.

Despite continued opposition from orthodox medicine, homeopathy is also making a modest comeback in the United States, where an estimated three thousand homeopaths—many of them also M.D.'s—now practice.

Is Less More?

Orthodox physicians react skeptically to homeopathy's Law of Similars, the idea that substances that cause certain symptoms cure the illnesses that cause the same symptoms. But they completely scoff at Hahnemann's other major tenet, the Law of Potentization, which says that homeopathic remedies become stronger as they become more dilute. Pharmacology says exactly the opposite. Critics charge that homeopathic remedies are so dilute that many contain *not even one molecule* of the active ingredient. Homeopaths counter that even without any of the active ingredient, super-dilute medicines retain a "healing essence." In 1938, the FDA granted homeopathic medicines over-the-counter status, based on the belief that such minute concentrations have no physiological effects at all—either adverse or beneficial. Critics say any benefits from homeopathic medicines are placebo effects.

Homeopaths grant that the Law of Potentization is counterintuitive and admit that they cannot explain how their medicines work. But they point to recent research showing that homeopathic microdoses have significant clinical benefit beyond placebo effects. For example, a 1980 double-blind study in the *British Journal of Clinical Pharmacology* showed that a homeopathic medicine significantly boosted the pain-relieving benefits of conventional drugs used to treat rheumatoid arthritis. And a 1986 double-blind study in *The Lancet* showed that a homeopathic preparation provided significant relief of allergy symptoms.

Homeopaths say one of orthodox medicine's most powerful tools, the vaccine, illustrates both the Law of Potentization and the Law of Similars. Vaccines are, in effect, very dilute microdoses of deactivated pathogens, toxins, or allergy-causing substances, which stimulate the immune system to marshal the body's defenses against the illness large doses of the active ingredient would cause. Many vaccines also cause temporary reactions which may mimic the symptoms of the conditions they are designed to prevent.

Homeopathic Cold Remedies

Although homeopaths recognize the common cold and flu as viral infections, they do not believe that viruses alone cause these illnesses. Like naturopaths, they view disease ecologically, saying that pathogens cause illness only when the host's immune system has been weakened enough to permit infection. The allopathic goal is to eliminate pathogens. Homeopaths strive to boost the immune response so that the body can heal itself.

Homeopathic medicines are packaged as tiny beads, with instructions that specify how many to place on the tongue and how often—usually three to six times a day. Because of their dilution, these remedies pose no overdose hazard when used as recommended. Even harsh critics concede that homeopathic medicines are nontoxic.

To be effective, the medicines must be matched as closely as possible to the symptoms the person is experiencing. Homeopaths describe symptoms more elaborately than orthodox physicians because minor differences in symptomatology might require a different medicine.

Space does not permit more than brief descriptions of cold symptoms and medicines. Those interested in pursuing homeopathic self-care should consult resources.

Homeopaths claim that if cold symptoms have been matched accurately with the right medicine, the cold should clear up after a night's rest. If not, try a different medicine. However, most homeopaths discourage the use of more than three medicines during any acute illness.

• *For colds with abrupt onset, fever, anxiety, and restlessness, take Aconite.* Aconite is a microdose of monkshood, which is highly toxic at large nonhomeopathic doses. *Do not* exceed the recommended dose. Sometimes called "homeopathic vitamin C," practitioners say it's most effective taken within twenty-four hours of the onset of cold symptoms.

• *For colds with abrupt onset, agitation, flushed face, watery nasal discharge, loss of mental sharpness, and possibly fever, take Belladonna.* Recall from chapter 11 that belladonna is a potentially deadly poison. *Do not* exceed the recommended dose. Microdoses of belladonna are used in some OTC cold formulas.

• *For colds characterized by sore throat and patchy, flushed face, without restlessness or loss of mental sharpness, take Ferrum phos.* Ferrum phos. is also known as ferric phosphate or white phosphate of iron.

• *For colds involving tearing eyes, burning nasal discharge, and frequent sneezing aggravated while indoors, in warm rooms, and in the evening, use Allium cepa. Allium cepa* is Latin for onion, a traditional cold remedy in large nonhomeopathic doses.

• *For colds with burning tears and nonirritating nasal discharge, which feel worse outdoors, in the morning and when lying down, try Euphrasia.* Euphrasia is a microdose of eyebright, a plant used since the Middle Ages to treat vision problems and other ailments, though sources dispute its safety and effectiveness in nonhomeopathic doses.

• *For late-stage colds with runny nose, thick stringy mucus, and possibly sinus headache, use Kali bichromium.* This medicine is also known as bichromate of potash.

• *For colds characterized by chest congestion, thirst, and coughing aggravated by talking or motion, take Byronia.* The common name for Byronia is wild hops, which is different from the hops used in brewing beer. Large, nonhomeopathic doses are toxic. *Do not* exceed the recommended dose.

• *For colds with thirst and nasal congestion that alternate with thick nasal discharge, with symptoms aggravated in warm rooms, try Pulsatilla.* This medicine is a microdose of windflower.

Those inexperienced in homeopathic self-care typically experience difficulty deciding which medicine to take. The materials in resources may help, but you might also obtain a homeopathic "combination formula" sold in some natural food stores. These preparations contain several of the medicines discussed above. Combination products may help, but most homeopaths say that they are not as effective as one properly chosen medicine.

Homeopathic medicines may be obtained by mail—see below.

RESOURCES

Everybody's Guide to Homeopathic Medicines by Stephen Cummings, F.N.P., and Dana Ullman, M.P.H., 1984, from J. P. Tarcher, Inc., Los Angeles; or available for $10.70 postpaid from Homeopathic Educational Services—see below.

Homeopathic Educational Services. 2124 Kittredge St. #Q, Berkeley, Calif. 94704; (415) 653-9270. The nation's largest distributor of homeopathic books, tapes, home medicine kits, and computer software. Publishes a national directory of four hundred practicing homeopaths.

Homeopathic Pharmacies: Boiron-Bornemann, 1208 Amosland Road, Norwood, Pa. 19074; (215) 532-2035; and Standard Homeopathic Pharmacy, 204 West 131st Street, Los Angeles, Calif. 90061; (213) 321-4284. Both publish extensive catalogs and sell homeopathic medicines by mail.

14

Promising New Cold Cures: Available Soon—and Now

The Girl Who Couldn't Swallow Her Medicine

In 1978 three-year-old Karen Eby, of Austin, Texas, was diagnosed with leukemia. She was placed on chemotherapy, but her father, George, an urban planner, wanted to do more—specifically, boost her suppressed immune system. Eby knew little about medicine, but his daughter's illness propelled him to the University of Texas Medical Library, where he studied leukemia and immunology. Eby found several studies showing that zinc stimulated T-cell activity. With the permission of Karen's physician, Eby gave his daughter zinc gluconate supplement tablets purchased at a natural food store.

Ordinarily, Karen swallowed her zinc tablets whole, but one day when she was coming down with a cold, her throat was so raw and inflamed she could not get the large tablets down and let one dissolve in her mouth instead. Colds are serious illnesses in those undergoing leukemia chemotherapy. They typically last two to three weeks. But a few hours after Karen sucked on the zinc, her family noticed that her cold symptoms had vanished.

Karen Eby's leukemia went into remission, but her father remained intrigued by her experience with zinc and continued to study the medical literature. Reports in the *Journal of Virology* and the British journal *Nature* showed that zinc interferes with rhinovirus replication.

At the first sign of a cold, Eby tried sucking on zinc gluconate lozenges himself, and his sore throats usually did not progress to full-blown colds. He urged his family and friends to try his cold cure, and they reported similar encouraging results.

The next step was a clinical trial. Eby quit his job, recruited Austin family practitioner William Halcomb, M.D., and University of Texas biochemist Donald Davis, Ph.D., and invested $10,000 of his own money to conduct a double-blind study. They gave 146 cold sufferers a supply of either zinc lozenges or a look-alike placebo. The subjects were instructed to let one lozenge dissolve in their mouths every two waking hours and not to take anything else for their colds. Compared to the placebo group, colds in the the zinc group cleared up an astonishing *seven days sooner.* Eby and his associates theorize that zinc coats the nasopharynx and inhibits viral replication.

Perhaps, but Felicia Geist and Judith Bateman, working in cold investigator Frederick Hayden's laboratory at the University of Virginia, pitted various concentrations of zinc gluconate and other zinc compounds against rhinoviruses in cell cultures and found no inhibition of viral replication. If zinc is a cold cure, Hayden says, it probably works by stimulating the immune system rather than attacking the virus directly.

The jury is still out on zinc, but Eby's work has spurred many people to take the mineral at the first sign of a cold, and quite a few report positive results. The FDA currently prohibits medicinal claims for zinc. However, it may be sold over-the-counter as a nutritional supplement, and a few companies hint at its newest use by marketing zinc pills "for the cold and flu season."

Zinc supplements (with zinc gluconate or zinc aspartate) are available at natural food stores. But the mineral has two problems—unpleasant taste and potential toxicity. Fortunately, several supplement manufacturers now market good-tasting candylike zinc lozenges made with orange or lemon flavoring and lots of sugar. The dose Eby recommends (23 milligrams) is 150 percent of the U.S. recommended daily allowance. Zinc is relatively safe, but those who take one lozenge every two hours might ingest eight lozenges a day, or 184 milligrams of zinc, which comes rather close to the dose that may cause adverse reactions (200 milligrams). If nausea, the first sign of zinc toxicity, develops, reduce dosage or stop taking the mineral. Zinc should not be taken for more than a few days. Cumulative toxicity is possible. In addition to nausea, long-term ingestion of high doses may cause vomiting, anemia, and lethargy.

Eby now holds a patent on zinc as a cold medicine. He has licensed it to "a major drug company" he declines to name and says the mineral is being tested for possible development as an OTC cold medication. The unnamed drug company has not yet filed a new drug application with the FDA, but Eby says he is optimistic about FDA approval by the early 1990s.

Interferon

Recall from chapter 3 that the immune system's T-cells release interferons, which spur the killer lymphocytes to attack cold virus particles and infected cells. Interferon, named for its ability to interfere with viral replication, was first isolated in 1957. Researchers immediately speculated that it might cure viral infections; unfortunately living organisms produce only vanishingly small amounts, and it seemed financially out of the question to recover enough for research purposes, let alone actual disease treatment.

Genetic engineering changed all that. By the early 1980s, all the interferons were available at a minute fraction of their original cost, and researchers have tested them against a broad range of illnesses from cancer to the common cold.

The early cold studies were discouraging. In 1984 two reports published simultaneously in the *Journal of Infectious Diseases* showed that alpha-interferon nasal spray reduced viral shedding during rhinovirus colds but was ineffective in preventing or treating them. In addition, up to two-thirds of those who used the interferon spray developed coldlike side effects: runny nose, nasal congestion, blood-tinged mucus, and nasal ulcerations. One set of authors concluded, "Interferon may not be useful in treating colds."

But in 1986, two studies published simultaneously in the *New England Journal of Medicine* resurrected alpha-interferon—this time as a cold preventive. Unlike the earlier treatment studies, in these it was provided to families who were instructed to use it preventively on healthy members whenever anyone else in the family developed a cold. Compared with the placebo group, the interferon-users suffered 30 to 40 percent fewer colds, and when nasal secretions were analyzed to identify the infecting virus, the interferon group contracted a whopping 80 percent fewer rhinovirus colds. In addition, the interferon spray was only half as concentrated as the formulation used in the earlier studies, and the rate of side effects dropped from more than 50 percent to just 12 percent. An editorial accompanying the studies hailed them as "remarkable. Short-term prophylaxis [cold prevention] with interferon may be practical."

There is no "may be" about it as far as Schering Corp. is concerned. In 1985, the Madison, New Jersey, pharmaceutical company, which supplied the researchers' interferon spray, filed a new drug application with the FDA to market the product under the brand-name Intron.

Intron is already licensed in Europe for cancer chemotherapy, where it costs $7.00 per million units. Family members in the successful interferon/cold studies each used 5 million units for seven days, or $245.00 per person per treatment course—to prevent less than half of all colds. Spokesmen for Schering-Plough say that if Intron wins FDA approval as a cold preventive, its price would be "lower."

Even if Intron's price drops, it would still be a prescription drug, necessitating the time and expense of a physician visit. Authorities predict that if the FDA approves it, Intron will be prescribed only to those at significant risk of serious cold complications: elderly or newborn hospital patients; those with severe asthma, cystic fibrosis, or other respiratory diseases; or those whose immune systems have been suppressed by cancer chemotherapy or drugs used to prevent organ-transplant rejection.

Spokespeople for the FDA and drug manufacturer decline to speculate when Intron might be approved. However, those familiar with the FDA licensing procedures say the process could take "years."

Several other antiviral drugs, notably enviroxime, have shown promise against cold viruses in test-tube studies, but human trials have been disappointing. The one exception seems to be WIN 51,711, developed by Sterling-Winthrop

Research Institute in Rensselaer, New York, which binds to rhinovirus particles and prevents them from injecting their genetic material into nasopharyngeal cells. It has been shown to work against thirty-two of thirty-three rhinoviruses in human cell cultures and against enterovirus infection in mice. Sterling-Winthrop plans to begin clinical trials "soon."

Block Those Receptors

The newest—and some say most exciting—cold cure of the future does not attack cold viruses at all. Instead, it uses genetically engineered proteins called *monoclonal antibodies* to occupy the receptor sites that rhinoviruses use to attach to nasopharyngeal cells. If the virus particles cannot "dock," they cannot cause infection.

This novel approach is the brainchild of Richard J. Colonno, Ph.D., a researcher at Merck, Sharp & Dohme pharmaceuticals in West Point, Pennsylvania. In the early 1980s, Colonno placed radioactive labels on twenty-four different rhinoviruses and tracked their paths into human cells. Twenty of the twenty-four attached to the same receptor site on the cells' membranes, which Colonno dubbed the "major" receptor. The other four all attached to a second site, the "minor" receptor. Colonno subsequently tested eighty-eight of the one hundred rhinoviruses and found that all of them use one of these two receptors. Colonno told the *Journal of the American Medical Association* that his work "reduces the problem of rhinovirus colds from trying to deal with 100 different viruses to trying to block only two receptors."

But as often happens in virology, blocking those two receptors turns out to be easier said than done. To develop a monoclonal antibody to occupy the major receptor, Colonno had to sift painstakingly through eight thousand cell cultures one by one. The task involved literally looking for a needle in a microscopic haystack. Colonno and associates examined thirteen cell cultures a day for sixty weeks until they found what they were looking for, in 1984. In laboratory tests, the elusive antibody outperformed Colonno's most optimistic expectations. "It has a very strong affinity for the major receptor, much higher than the viruses'. You can prebind virus particles to cells, add antibody, and show that the antibody *displaces* the virus. Something that strong is capable of literally stopping a cold dead in its tracks."

In early 1986, Colonno arranged a clinical trial in association with University of Virginia cold researchers Hayden and Gwaltney. Thirteen volunteers used nasal spray containing the monoclonal antibody, and thirteen controls used a placebo. Then both groups were inoculated with rhinovirus 39, which binds to the major receptor. Unfortunately, every subject in both groups caught the cold. But significantly, those in the antibody group developed their colds one or two days later and experienced milder symptoms, which suggests that Colonno may be on the right track.

Colonno is searching for an antibody to occupy the minor site and trying to reduce the molecular size of his major-site antibody to reduce the likelihood of undesired immune system reactions.

Cold researchers express cautious excitement about Colonno's work. His discovery of the two rhinovirus-receptor sites is clearly important, and his studies to date have been intriguing. But there are millions of receptors in the nose, and it takes very few virus particles to cause a cold. To work effectively, Colonno's antibody must achieve an extremely—some say impossibly—high degree of receptor coverage.

Colonno says he hopes to have "some kind of solid lead" by 1990. If he does, a monoclonal antibody rhinovirus cold cure might be available by the mid-1990s.

RESOURCE

Good-tasting zinc lozenges. The most widely distributed is "Cold Season Plus" from Quantum Research, Inc., P.O. Box 2791, Eugene, Or. 97401; 1-(800)-448-1448, in Oregon (503) 345-5556. Several flavors are available. Each contains 23 mg of elemental zinc in a base of fruit sugar (fructose) with 150 mg of vitamin C, 1,000 I.U. of vitamin A, and three herbs: propolis, slippery elm, and goldenseal (see chapter 11). Sold at natural food stores and some pharmacies.

15

Playing It Safe While Pregnant and Nursing

Until the early 1960s, most physicians believed that drugs taken by pregnant women could not cross the placenta and harm the developing fetus. Then came Thalidomide, a sleep aid sold over-the-counter in Europe from 1957 to 1961. Thalidomide was quite popular—until it was shown to cause serious limb malformations in an estimated eight thousand children whose mothers took it while pregnant. The ensuing scandal spurred the adoption of stricter drug-licensing regulations on both sides of the Atlantic and persuaded physicians that the so-called "placental barrier" did not exist.

Since then we've learned that virtually all drugs cross the placenta and reach the fetus. However, 85 percent of drugs currently in use have never been tested for safety during pregnancy on laboratory animals. No pharmacologically active compound has ever been shown to be entirely harmless to human fetuses in all stages of pregnancy. Therefore, authorities urge pregnant women to *avoid all drugs not prescribed by their physicians.* But studies show that through the early 1980s as many as *half* of all pregnant women used OTC drugs, including many cold formulas and herbs whose ingredients have been associated with increased risks of miscarriage and birth defects.

No cold remedy causes problems in all pregnancies. Drug effects on the fetus depend on dosage, genetic susceptibility, length of exposure, and stage of pregnancy. The higher the dose, the longer the exposure, and the earlier in the pregnancy, the greater the risk of harm. But why take chances? Colds almost always clear up within two weeks without any drug treatment whatsoever. And nondrug alternatives often help a great deal—see "Safe Cold Remedies During Pregnancy," below.

Beware of These Drugs

Pregnant women should avoid *all* pharmacologically active cold remedies, but the following deserve special mention:

• *Alcohol.* Most liquid cold formulas contain alcohol. Heavy use is associated with serious physical and mental defects known as fetal alcohol syndrome. The U.S. surgeon general and most physicians urge pregnant women not to drink at all.
• *Antihistamines.* Common in multisymptom cold formulas. Even though physicians may prescribe them to women with serious allergies, antihistamines are associated with an increased risk of birth defects in animal studies.
• *Aspirin.* An ingredient in many OTC cold formulas, aspirin is associated with an increased risk of birth defects in laboratory animals. Large amounts may cause miscar-

riage. Frequent use toward the end of pregnancy may cause fetal hemorrhaging.

• *Caffeine.* Common in OTC cold formulas. In laboratory animals, large doses are associated with miscarriage, stillbirth, premature labor, and birth defects. Caffeine also raises blood pressure. Approximately 5 percent of pregnant women develop pregnancy-related high blood pressure, known as preeclampsia or toxemia of pregnancy. Anyone with preeclampsia should avoid caffeine. Other pregnant women are advised to limit their daily intake to one cup of coffee, or two cans of cola, or three cups of black tea.

• *Decongestants.* Many OTC cold formulas contain decongestants. Like caffeine, they also raise blood pressure. Women with preeclampsia should not use them.

Beware of These Herbs

• *Angelica.* Large doses may cause miscarriage.
• *Cayenne.* Large doses may cause nausea and vomiting. Women troubled by morning sickness should use small doses or avoid it.
• *Coltsfoot.* Contains carcinogens.
• *Comfrey.* Contains carcinogens.
• *Elder.* Large doses may cause nausea and vomiting.
• *Ephedra.* Elevates blood pressure. Women with preeclampsia should not use it.
• *Horehound.* Large doses may cause nausea and vomiting.
• *Licorice.* Elevates blood pressure.

Beware of Acupressure

Pregnant women—especially those in the third trimester—should avoid acupressure because several points may stimulate uterine contractions and cause premature labor.

Safe Cold Remedies During Pregnancy

Most of these self-treatments are discussed in greater detail in chapter 8:

- *Sore throat.* Suck on hard candies or gargle with warm salt water.
- *Headache.* Lie down, or take a bath or shower, or try cool, moist towels on your face and forehead, or get a neck and shoulder massage.
- *Fever.* Consult your physician immediately. Prolonged fevers over 100° F may harm the fetus. In such cases, most physicians advise a short course of acetaminophen. Acetaminophen may not be 100 percent safe, but for fever during pregnancy, most physicians believe that the benefits outweigh the risks.
- *Lethargy.* Lie down. Take frequent naps.
- *Runny nose.* Use disposable tissues. If your nose or upper lip become irritated, use a moisturizing skin lotion.
- *Congestion.* Try a vaporizer, hot bath, or shower; warm, moist towels on your face; or drink hot chicken soup or other hot fluids. At night use extra pillows.
- *Dry cough.* Try a vaporizer, hot bath, or shower, or suck on hard candies.

While Nursing

Just as drugs cross the placenta, they also contaminate the nursing mother's milk. Once the baby is born, of course, maternal drug use can no longer cause birth defects, but most authorities urge nursing mothers to observe the same precautions as pregnant women. When in doubt, consult your physician.

16

Cold Cures for Children

Most children suffer colds "10 times as often as all other illnesses combined," according to the current edition of *Baby and Child Care* by the venerable Dr. Benjamin Spock. A recent study shows that about one-third of young children are sick at any given time, mostly with colds. Childhood colds account for an estimated 20 percent of all pediatrician visits, and cold complications—primarily ear infection, strep throat, and persistent cough—account for 25 to 40 percent more.

One of the primary tasks of early childhood is to exercise the developing immune system by confronting the more than two hundred cold viruses. Five of the six families of cold viruses strike children more frequently than adults and linger longer. By age two, the typical child has suffered twelve to twenty colds involving the full range of symptoms and probably as many that produce either no symptoms or just a runny nose.

Since colds are spread by close contact, children suffer colds in proportion to the number of other children in their lives and the amount of time spent with them. Most parents report a significant increase in colds if children are placed in large-population day-care facilities and a noticeable decrease if they are removed to day care involving only one or two other children.

Children also shed virus (remain infective) far longer than adults. People of all ages begin to shed virus twelve to forty-eight hours before their first symptoms appear. Adult shedding peaks on day three, then subsides quickly. But children may shed virus for up to several weeks, prompting authorities to estimate that kids in day care and nursery school are either infected or capable of infecting others up to half the time.

Colds are rarely serious in children. Most can be treated effectively at home with telephone backup from one's pediatrician or family practitioner. Nonetheless, parents should be alert for the symptoms of potentially serious cold complications: ear infection, asthma attacks, croup, and lower respiratory infections, such as bronchiolitis, bronchitis, and pneumonia (see chapter 17). They should also learn how to distinguish the common cold from the "cold counterfeits," possibly serious illnesses that begin with coldlike symptoms: flu, strep throat, tonsillitis, whooping cough, mumps, meningitis, and several other diseases (see chapter 18).

How to

Childhood colds may be treated with any of the healing arts already discussed—orthodox medicine, vitamin C, chicken soup, acupressure, homeopathy, zinc, or herbs—but with several important caveats:

• *Manage children's colds in consultation with your pediatrician or family practitioner.* Cold complications and counterfeits are much more likely in children than adults. Some may be serious. When in doubt, call the child's physician. Most orthodox doctors look askance at alternative healing arts. If you are interested in these therapies, either look for a physician familiar with them (many homeopaths and acupuncturists are also M.D.'s), or consult an alternative practitioner in addition to your physician.

• *Use all cold remedies conservatively.* It's one thing to experiment on yourself, quite another to do so on your children. Many cold remedies—pharmaceutical and herbal—are not recommended for infants. In addition, young children may choke on pills. Either crush and mix them with food or give liquid medicines (Dimetapp is one brand). Adjust all dosages downward to reflect children's lower body weights. OTCs specify children's doses, but it's wise to consult your physician or pharmacist for infant and toddler dosages. Some Chinese herb preparations specify children's dosages, but others do not. When in doubt, consult a Chinese physician or one of the Chinese pharmacies mentioned in chapter 12.

The microdoses used in homeopathic medicines are considered safe for all ages, but homeopaths say they often act faster in children than adults. When in doubt, consult a homeopath or one of the homeopathic pharmacies mentioned in chapter 13.

Be especially conservative when giving alcohol and bulk herbal teas to children. Most authorities discourage any alcohol use by children, and as discussed in chapter 11, bulk herbs have inherent dose-control problems. If you give your children herb teas, dilute them, and beware of the aromatic herbs (for example, peppermint) which may trigger choking.

Many medications have exaggerated—and sometimes paradoxical—effects on children. Since the vast majority of colds clear up without any treatment, and since non-drug approaches often provide equal—or superior—relief, the rule of thumb for administering cold medications to children is: When in doubt, don't.

• *Learn the symptoms of cold complications and counterfeits.* These are discussed more fully in chapters 17 and 18. However, seek medical attention immediately if the child

Suffers difficult, labored, or rapid breathing
Becomes markedly irritable, lethargic, or complains of a stiff neck
Suffers any seizure

Call your physician if the child

Tugs on an ear
Develops any rash
Has bloody sputum or stool
Develops any of the fever signs discussed in the "Fever" section below

• *Make sure the child gets adequate rest.* Confinement to bed is rarely necessary, but if possible, the child should stay at home while symptoms persist in order to prevent infecting others. Some medical centers now offer special day-care facilities for sick kids or programs that send nursing aides to the homes of sick children so that their parents can go to work.

• *If any adults in the house smoke, they should stop.* Over and above risking their own health, exposure to smoke aggravates childhood respiratory problems.

• *Make sure the child drinks plenty of fluids.* Adequate hydration is more important for cold-infected children than for adults because kids are more susceptible to dehydration from fever. Childhood colds are more likely to cause fever, and children have greater surface-to-volume ratios, hence they lose proportionately more moisture through perspiration. Warm fluids clear nasal mucus better than cold fluids, but *all* fluids help prevent dehydration. (Milk may not be a good idea for children prone to ear infections—see "Earache," below. Use water or juice.)

For specific cold symptoms in children:

• *Sore throat.* Try a vaporizer, warm liquids with honey, lemon, and perhaps a tiny pinch of licorice root, or the Ho-Ku acupressure point discussed in chapter 12. Children over four or five may suck on hard candies or medicated sore-throat lozenges; younger children might choke. Acetaminophen may also help relieve pain—see below for dosage.

• *Fever.* Unlike most adult colds, childhood upper respiratory infections frequently cause fever. Recall from chapter 3 that fever is one of the immune system's defenses against viral infection. Low-grade fevers need not be treated unless the child seems uncomfortable. If so, try the Ta-Chui or Chu-Chih acupressure points, a sponge bath, or acetaminophen. Sponging encourages evaporation, which may reduce body temperature (although recent research has questioned its value). Higher fevers should be treated with acetaminophen. It may be given every four to six hours. Consult your physician or pharmacist for dosage, but the following are often recommended:

Infants to eleven pounds, 40 milligrams.
Infants eleven to seventeen pounds, 80 milligrams.
Toddlers to twenty-three pounds, 120 milligrams.
Toddlers twenty-three to thirty-five pounds, 160 milligrams.
Preschoolers to fifty pounds, 240 milligrams.

Elementary school children, 320 to 400 milligrams.
Adolescents, 480 milligrams.

• *Do not give aspirin to children under eighteen for colds, flu, and chicken pox.* Aspirin is associated with Reye's syndrome, a rare but frequently fatal condition that affects the brain, liver, and kidneys. The federal Centers for Disease Control (CDC) in Atlanta recorded ninety-one cases around the country in 1985. Twenty-eight (32 percent) of these children died. In 1985 half of Reye's syndrome cases occurred in January and February, and half in children under four. Fortunately, publicity of the aspirin/Reye's link has resulted in a major shift to acetaminophen in recent years, and the incidence of Reye's syndrome has fallen 66 percent since 1981.

Although most childhood fevers can be treated at home, call the child's physician immediately for any fever

In an infant less than four weeks old.
Over 101°F in an infant less than three months.
Over 102°F.
That resists treatment for two days.
That begins in the middle of a cold.
That subsides, then returns a few days later.
With any rash.
With marked irritability, confusion, stiff neck, or loss of consciousness.

Children may develop high fevers quite rapidly, and some occasionally suffer "fever fits" (febrile seizures) which terrify parents. Three to 5 percent of normal, healthy children have at least one febrile seizure. They have nothing to do with epilepsy or other neurological disorders. Febrile seizures develop when a rapid increase in body temperature causes electrical impulses from the brain to misfire, resulting in the eyes rolling back, convulsions or rhythmic beating of one or more limbs, and possible vomiting, urination, or defecation. Fortunately, febrile seizures usually last no more than five minutes (five of the longest minutes of a parent's life). Fewer than half the children who suffer one febrile seizure have a second, and fewer than half of those experience a third. Although a seizing child is a terrifying sight, febrile seizures rarely cause lasting health problems. During a febrile seizure, place the child facedown in bed, head turned to one side, and protected from hitting anything hard. Don't force anything into the child's mouth to prevent tongue biting or swallowing; these occur very rarely in febrile seizures. Make sure the child can breathe freely by clearing any vomitus from the nose and mouth. Sponge the child for the fever reduction it may promote and to provide the reassurance of parental touch. After the seizure, the child may be groggy or temporarily weak. Consult your physician immediately for a postseizure evaluation. If a fever is high enough to cause a seizure, there's a possibility of meningitis.

• *Runny nose.* Try disposable tissues, a vaporizer, or the Ying-Hsiang acupressure point (see chapter 12). (When measuring half a thumb width from the nostril, use the child's thumb, not yours.) Runny nose is the leading physical symptom in infants and toddlers. It is one of the more tolerable—if not attractive—cold symptoms. Physicians generally recommend no treatment unless the child becomes noticeably uncomfortable. A more aggressive nondrug approach uses a nasal syringe to suck out excess mucus. If you must give the child medication, try a children's OTC antihistamine/decongestant combination. Consult your pharmacist or physician for dosage.
• *Nasal congestion.* Try a vaporizer, chicken soup, other hot fluids, aromatic chest rub, or any of the several acupressure points recommended for colds. A nasal syringe

may also help. At night prop the child's head up on extra pillows. However, if the child becomes uncomfortable or develops noisy breathing, decongestant nose drops may be indicated. Decongestants have the same problem in children as in adults—rebound congestion from overuse (more than every three or four hours for more than three days). The major side effect of oral decongestants is insomnia, so don't administer them too late in the day.

• *Earache.* Ear inflammation is a typical cold symptom in children under four. Ear pain is caused by a buildup of fluid pressure in the middle ear, the area behind the eardrum. This fluid usually drains into the nasopharynx through the eustachian tube, but during a cold the tube may become constricted or shut, causing fluid backup, pressure, and pain. Earaches are prevalent in young children because their eustachian tubes are quite narrow. The child with ear pain cries seemingly inconsolably and pulls or rubs the ear. To prevent ear complications, make sure the child's head is elevated at night and during naps to promote fluid drainage. And don't give kids with colds bottles of milk in bed. Some studies suggest that drinking milk while lying down promotes ear irritation. To relieve childhood ear pain, use a heating pad, acetaminophen, anesthetic ear drops, or warm vegetable-oil ear drops. Some cold-related earaches become ear infections (see chapter 17).

• *Cough.* For uncomplicated dry coughs due to colds, use a vaporizer, hard candies, or the Chih-Tse acupressure point (see chapter 12), and encourage the child to drink plenty of warm fluids. An aromatic chest rub might help, but may also cause skin irritation. A children's cough suppressant with dextromethorphan may provide additional relief, especially at night. Consult the packaging, your pharmacist, or physician for dosage. In some cases, a physician might prescribe codeine.

One final note: Although most children's colds may be

treated at home, sometimes when physician visits are really necessary, parents hesitate to bring them in for fear of exposing them to other children who may have more serious communicable illnesses. Although flu and other illnesses may be transmitted in waiting rooms, a recent study in the *New England Journal of Medicine* suggests that as a rule, this is not a major problem. Investigators studied 127 healthy children aged six months to three years who saw their physicians for checkups. In the week afterward, 38 percent of them got sick. In a control group of kids who did not visit their pediatricians, 40 percent became ill, a statistically insignificant difference.

17

Cold Complications: Beyond a Week of Congestion

Sometimes the common cold consumes so much of the immune system's energy that cold viruses, other viruses, or bacteria, breach the respiratory tract's remaining defenses and cause secondary infections, or complications. Cold complications occur most frequently—and tend to be most severe—in infants, the elderly, and the chronically ill, but they may also strike otherwise healthy children and adults. One cold complication, pneumonia, may become quite serious—possibly even fatal for those in the risk groups mentioned.

Ear Infection

Ear infection (otitis media) is by far the leading cold complication in children, accounting for an estimated 25 percent of all pediatrician visits. Ear infections, which usually strike children six months to four years, often cause the sharpest, most persistent pain infants and children have ever felt. Parents must cope not only with screaming offspring, but also with their own fears about what is often an infant's first significant illness.

As discussed in the "Earache" section of chapter 16, upper respiratory infections often constrict the eustachian tubes that normally drain secretions into the nasopharynx from the middle ear. Impaired drainage traps fluid in the middle ear. As fluid pressure increases, so does pain. If viruses or bacteria climb up the eustachian tubes, the trapped fluid becomes infected. As ear infection progresses, the immune system sends additional fluid and white blood cells to the middle ear, aggravating pressure and pain. The classic ear infection involves fever, seemingly inconsolable crying, and rubbing or pulling on the affected ear(s).

About 70 percent of ear infections are caused by bacteria, but even when they are viral, a secondary bacterial infection may develop, which is why the standard treatment is an antibiotic—with acetaminophen for pain. Studies show that ampicillin works best, but if the child has not improved within a day or two, the physician may prescribe amoxicillin, erythromycin, penicillin, or sulfa drugs.

Although ear infections may respond rapidly to antibiotics and clear up entirely within a day or two, it's important to give the child the full ten-day course of medication to kill *all* the bacteria, including the small number that may be relatively resistant. This helps prevent recurrences and further complications, such as mastoiditis, or hearing impairment. In addition to killing harmful bacteria, antibiotics also kill the beneficial bacteria that populate the intestines and help in food digestion. Unless these good bacteria are replenished, antibiotic users may suffer diarrhea or intestinal upset. There are two ways to replenish these beneficial bacteria—eat yogurt or take lactobacillus capsules. Yogurt is best for children.

Antihistamines are ineffective against ear infections, and decongestants are controversial. Some physicians prescribe decongestants—and many herbals recommend ephedra (one teaspoon of tea three times a day)—to help open narrowed eustachian tubes and promote drainage. Those who favor decongestants sometimes suggest starting treatment at the first sign of a cold as a preventive. However, other authorities say that decongestant benefits, if any, are not worth the risks: insomnia from pills (and ephedra teas) and rebound congestion from sprays. Parents must decide for themselves after consulting with their children's physicians.

Some parents find that ear infections are less likely to develop if, at the first sign of a cold, they eliminate from their children's diet foods often associated with allergic reactions: animal and dairy products, wheat, corn, and sweeteners, and limit the child's diet to fresh fruits and vegetables, non-wheat and -corn cereals, and juices.

Studies show that bottle-fed babies are more susceptible to ear infections than breast-fed babies, particularly those who take bottles while lying down.

Severe recurrent ear infections may contribute to hearing impairment, language-acquisition difficulties, and learning disabilities. Fears of these problems and the trauma of chronically sick children sometimes drive parents to seek more aggressive treatment. Surgical treatment (tympanostomy) punctures the eardrums and inserts small drainage tubes into the child's middle ears. Although this approach provides immediate relief, it is quite controversial. The tubes may provide a path for pathogens *into* the middle ear, or the tubes might fall out, requiring additional surgery, with added risk of ear damage.

Parents interested in spending less time and money on physician and emergency-room visits for ear infections might consider purchasing an otoscope, the instrument physicians use to examine the ears (see resources). Studies show that as parents become more familiar with ear examination, they feel less victimized by this common cold complication. Parents who learn to examine their children's ears can distinguish between earaches and ear infections, often preventing unnecessary anxiety and physician visits.

Bronchiolitis

The small airways in infants' lungs (bronchioles) are much narrower than those in older children or adults. If they become infected, typically after winter colds caused by respiratory syncytial virus or one of the parainfluenza viruses, the result is bronchiolitis, which causes rapid breathing with prolonged, labored exhalations, fever, and anxiety in children from birth to two years. Bronchiolitis typically lasts from four to ten days. It is rarely serious unless it develops in children who are hospitalized or chronically ill.

Until recently, treatment involved rest; acetaminophen; liquids; humidification with a vaporizer, teakettle, or hot shower; and parental cuddling to help relieve anxiety. Now an effective antiviral drug, ribavirin (Virazole), may be prescribed. Since bronchiolitis is a viral illness, antibiotics are ineffective, though they may be prescribed if bacterial complications develop.

Some studies suggest that infants who develop bronchiolitis are at increased risk for asthma.

Croup

The term *croup* comes from the old Scottish word *roup,* which means "hoarse cry." Croup typically strikes infants and children six months to three years old. The major symptoms are a high-pitched sound on inhalation ("stridor") then a "barking" cough, which often begins at night toward the end of a cold or flu. Other possible symptoms include fever and rapid breathing. Most cases occur in the fall or winter and more often in boys than in girls. Acetaminophen and humidification usually relieve most cases within a day. Persistent croup may require hospitalization and administration of oxygen though a face mask or "croup tent."

Asthma Attacks

An estimated 3 percent of children under seventeen have asthma, characterized by bronchial spasms, cough, and wheezing (high-pitched exhalation), which may be severe. Asthma is the leading cause of childhood hospitalization in the United States. Attacks may be triggered by tobacco smoke; chemical fumes; strenuous exercise; allergies to pollen, dander, and foods; or upper respiratory infections. Emotional stress may aggravate attacks. The cause of asthma remains a mystery, but it often runs in families and is more common in boys than in girls. Children with a history of bronchiolitis are at increased risk. Any child who develops wheezing or labored breathing during or shortly after a cold or flu should be evaluated by a physician. Asthma can usually be controlled with a combination of parent-and-child education; relaxation and breathing exercises; self-monitoring of respiratory function using a peak flow monitor (see resources); moderate physical exercise, particularly yoga, which has been shown to be remarkably effective; and in severe cases, a variety of medications (epinephrine, inhaled bronchodilators, and cromolyn sodium). About half of asthma sufferers' attacks cease after their teens.

Tonsillitis

The tonsils are lymph glands on either side of the upper throat. They are large in infants, then shrink throughout childhood until they become approximately almond-sized by adulthood. The tonsils filter disease organisms out of the mouth and throat before they can cause illness. But sometimes virus particles or bacteria overwhelm the tonsils, and they become infected, inflamed, and enlarged, causing sore throat, painful swallowing, and possibly fever. Physicians typically culture a swab from the tonsil area, and if bacteria grow, prescribe an antibiotic—and rest, fluids, warm saltwater gargles, and acetaminophen. Viral tonsillitis is treated the same way, minus the antibiotic. The infection usually clears up in a few days to a week (but if antibiotics are prescribed, be sure to take the entire course). In children, infected tonsils occasionally become so enlarged that they partially block drainage from the eustachian tubes, causing an ear infection as well. Surgical tonsil removal (tonsillectomy) was once almost routine for children who developed tonsillitis or a variety of other conditions, including frequent colds. During the 1950s and 1960s, an estimated 1 million children a year had tonsillectomies. Today this operation is performed only if a child has several attacks of strep-positive tonsillitis with fever.

Sinus Infection

The sinuses are hollow, air-filled, mucus-lined areas in the bones of the face around the nose and eyes that give the voice its resonance. Although sinus infections (sinusitis) usually develop as complications of colds or flu, this disease is typically bacterial. Facial pain around the nose and eyes distinguishes sinusitis from colds and flu. Other symptoms include headache, runny nose, tearing, and possibly fever. Home treatments include decongestants, fluids, saltwater nose drops, analgesics, and humidification. Physicians typically prescribe antibiotics. Facial acupressure and herbal decongestant teas may also help.

Bronchitis

Many people develop lingering, annoying, productive, or nonproductive coughs toward the end of many of their colds. Bronchitis can strike anyone, but it is associated with a history of asthma and/or allergies, exposure to tobacco smoke or chemical fumes, and dry environments, such as homes with forced-air heating. If fever and chest pain accompany any cough, see a physician promptly to rule out pneumonia. But for a lingering cold-related cough without fever, use humidification, dextromethorphan, acupressure, an herbal cough suppressant, hard candies, or medicated cough drops. Nonsmokers tend to develop the nonproductive cough. Bronchitis in smokers is often productive, may be chronic, and may respond to antibiotics.

Pneumonia

A generic term for any lung infection, pneumonia is the most severe—sometimes fatal—complication of the common cold and flu. Caused by viruses, bacteria, fungi, or other microorganisms, pneumonia floods the tiny air sacs of the lungs with fluid, resulting in high fever, shaking chills, chest pain, difficult breathing, and a dry cough that progresses to a productive cough often yielding rust-colored (blood-tinged) sputum. Smoking and alcoholism increase risk substantially. Pneumonia typically occurs toward the end of the upper respiratory infection. The person's fever (if any) has subsided and recovery appears to be progressing—then a high fever and other pneumonia symptoms develop. *If pneumonia symptoms appear, see a physician immediately.* Most cases in otherwise healthy children or adults are relatively mild and can be treated with rest, fluids, acetaminophen, and antibiotics if culturing shows bacteria. But pneumonia may become serious—and demands immediate medical attention.

Cold Sores/Fever Blisters

These red, crusty, open sores, which typically erupt on or near the lips in association with colds or flu, are caused by the herpes simplex virus type-1 (HSV-I), similar to the one that causes genital herpes (HSV-II). By age fourteen, an estimated 70 percent of Americans have antibodies to HSV-I, which means that they have been exposed—typically by kissing. However, only a fraction of those who have been infected ever develop the characteristic skin eruptions, and even fewer suffer recurrences with subsequent colds and flu. HSV-I is highly contagious. The virus sheds from the sores and, in recurring cases, from the areas where they develop during the period a day or two before the sore appears ("prodrome"). Those who have recurrent cold sores should learn how their prodromes feel—a slight tingling is common—and refrain from kissing and oral/genital contact until their sores are completely healed, usually in seven to ten days. The initial outbreak tends to be the most painful. An ice pack applied for an hour or two to the emerging recurrent cold sore may prevent the eruption. Acyclovir, a recently developed prescription drug available in ointment form, may also be used.

RESOURCES

Earscope. For less than the cost of one office visit, this professional-style otoscope allows parents to examine their children's ears and diagnose and treat incipient infections before they become more advanced and traumatic. Includes instructions and "A Parent's Guide to Childhood Ear Infections," reprinted from *Medical Self-Care.* Contact the *Self-Care Catalog,* 11 Chapel St., Augusta, Me. 04330; (207) 622-5949.

Asthma Alert Kit. Contains a peak-flow monitor, which measures exhalation force. Decreased peak flow may signal an impending asthma attack before it occurs, allowing parents and children to take preventive or treatment steps before wheezing—and anxieties—begin. Includes instructions, charting materials, and "Asthma: A Breath of Fresh Air" reprinted from *Medical Self-Care.* Contact the *Self-Care Catalog,* address above.

CHAPTER
18

Cold Counterfeits: Influenza and Other Look-Alikes

Many illnesses—some potentially serious—begin with symptoms that may be mistaken for the common cold. Those committed to self-care should become familiar with the "cold counterfeits" because some demand immediate medical attention.

Influenza (Flu)

Like the common cold, influenza is a viral infection of the upper respiratory tract. In the classic case, you feel fine, then suddenly develop a headache. On your way to the medicine cabinet, you feel a little achy and wonder if you're catching a cold. Moments later, you suddenly feel *terrible*. You have a temperature of 101°, and can barely crawl into bed, where you remain feverish and weak for several days. You're sicker than you've felt in years. You have no appetite and barely enough strength to go to the bathroom.

When flu strikes, most people treat it like a bad cold. But the combination of flu and its chief complication, pneumonia, is the nation's *fifth leading cause of death,* claiming more than fifty thousand lives each year—and periodically many more. Fortunately, the most serious type of flu can usually be prevented with a vaccine, or treated effectively with a safe prescription drug.

Several times each century, the influenza virus undergoes significant genetic change, and instead of the local epidemics we usually experience each winter, a worldwide epidemic, or "pandemic," occurs. Hippocrates recorded one that swept the Mediterranean in 412 B.C. Medical historians have deduced that there have been pandemics approximately every thirty to fifty years, including those of 1781, 1830, and 1889, which swept across Russia and Europe from Asia. During the Middle Ages, physicians believed that influenza was celestial in origin, "a blast from the stars." The term *influenza* is derived from the Italian, *influentia coeli,* meaning "celestial influence."

The worst pandemic this century, the Spanish flu of 1918–19, infected half the world's population in three increasingly virulent waves, and killed 20 million people—sixty-five thousand in the United States—including many healthy people of all ages. An estimated 80 percent of U.S. Army deaths during World War I were caused not by enemy fire but by the Spanish flu. In fact, many historians say that this flu may have cost Germany the war. The German army was so decimated by the disease that General Erich von Ludendorff's army along the Marne could barely fight.

In 1957, 40 million Americans fell ill with Asian flu, which contributed to seventy thousand deaths. During the epidemic of Hong Kong flu in 1968–69, fifty-six thousand Americans died. Epidemiologists do not rule out the possibility of a future pandemic like the one in 1918.

Unlike the common cold, which infects only humans and a few species of monkeys, influenza also infects—and is transmissible to humans by—pigs, horses, seals, and a large number of birds. A few years ago, a strain similar to the 1918 flu was discovered in turkeys in Pennsylvania. Because of the danger to the human population, public health officials insisted that poultry farmers destroy 17 million infected birds.

Flu symptoms include headache, fever, sore throat, nasal congestion, runny nose, and cough. Children may suffer diarrhea. Sometimes it's difficult to tell the difference between the flu and the common cold. If an upper respiratory infection hits you like a truck with sudden fever, body aches, and weakness bordering on physical collapse that sends you right to bed, it's probably flu. Unfortunately, flu symptoms can be quite variable. Not everyone feels forced into bed. For some, the only symptom that distinguishes the flu from a cold is the sudden fever. In other cases, it's the headache and body aches. And in some, there are no differences at all.

The variability of flu symptoms is due, in part, to the fact that there are three types of influenza—designated A, B, and C. Type-A flu (also known as influenza A) is the most serious. It usually (but not always) produces the sudden high fever, physical collapse, and body aches that are the hallmarks of classic flu. Influenza A is responsible for many annual flu epidemics, and the periodic pandemics.

Influenza B may also cause sudden fever, weakness, and body aches, but its symptoms are typically less severe and don't last as long. Type-B flu feels more like a cold. Like influenza A, type-B flu can cause epidemics, but unlike its viral relative, influenza B outbreaks tend to remain localized and do not become pandemics.

Influenza C is hardly even an illness. It causes only minor coldlike symptoms in children—mild fever, nasal congestion, and runny nose—and is not considered a public health problem. Type-C flu rarely causes illness in adults. When public health officials say "flu," they mean influenza A or B.

Although colds may cause a variety of complications, the most severe, pneumonia, is rare, even among the usual risk groups. Influenza A, on the other hand, is much more likely to cause pneumonia. The risk of this potentially fatal complication makes it important to know whether any upper respiratory infection during midwinter flu season is, in fact, influenza. Unfortunately, flu symptoms can be so varied that without sophisticated laboratory equipment, it's often impossible to tell.

That's why the CDC carefully tracks influenza outbreaks in the United States and around the world. During flu season, from December through April, the CDC Influenza Branch issues frequent flu bulletins to public health officials and the news media. Flu information may also be obtained from physicians or the Infectious Disease Office of local health departments.

Influenza spreads primarily by the aerosol route. A 1979 report in the *American Journal of Epidemiology* describes how an airline passenger with influenza A infected 72 percent of fellow travelers within four hours, including the plane's cockpit crew, who had no direct contact with the flu sufferer. The virus spread through the jet's air-conditioning system. Flu also spreads much faster than most cold viruses, especially if the infected are heavy coughers.

Like the common cold, people infected with flu shed virus before they develop any symptoms and continue to shed for several days after the fever subsides. Children may shed virus for up to two weeks. Authorities believe that children in close contact in school during the fall months provide the breeding ground for the nation's flu outbreaks each winter.

You don't even have to get sick to spread influenza. Many people who develop antibodies—proving that they were exposed—show no symptoms, or only very mild cold-like symptoms. But they may still spread the virus to others, who might suffer severe illness.

The CDC calls annual vaccination "the single most important measure" against influenza. Because flu viruses undergo frequent genetic changes, a new vaccine is developed each year, which protects against every strain of influenza A and B active around the world the previous flu season. Flu vaccine is available from physicians and most public health departments, many of which provide it free to those at risk—for example, nursing-home residents and staff.

Anyone can get vaccinated, even pregnant women after their first trimester. But those at risk *definitely should:* those over sixty-five and anyone over six months with respiratory diseases, heart disease, diabetes, or other chronic illnesses.

Although flu can strike year-round, major annual outbreaks usually occur during winter and early spring. It takes about two weeks after vaccination to develop effective immunity, so authorities recommend immunization from late October through November.

There are two kinds of flu vaccine, both equally effective. One is made from deactivated whole virus; the other uses only part of it ("split virus"). The CDC recommends the split-virus vaccine for children up to age twelve because it causes fewer side effects in young people than the whole-virus vaccine, which is recommended for everyone else.

Public health authorities call flu vaccine side effects "quite mild." About 25 percent of recipients experience some short-term soreness at the injection site. Five to 10 percent feel a little achy, and report mild cold symptoms. Children may develop a low-grade fever for a day or two, though the likelihood is minimized with the split-virus vaccine. Serious reactions are almost unheard of except for people who are allergic to eggs (used to manufacture the vaccine); these people should not get vaccinated. For everyone else, flu vaccine's benefits greatly outweigh its risks.

Despite flu vaccine's safety, the CDC estimates that only 20 percent of Americans at risk for influenza-related complications get vaccinated each year. "Most people just don't see influenza as serious enough to warrant the special trip," says Dr. Karl Kappus of the CDC Influenza Branch. "Many physicians don't encourage vaccination. And flu vaccine has a lingering—completely undeserved—bad reputation because of what happened with swine flu."

The 1976 swine flu virus bore striking resemblance to the strain that caused the killer pandemic of 1918. Worried health officials rushed to produce a vaccine, then mounted a huge campaign to get the country vaccinated. For reasons that remain a mystery, the feared pandemic never materialized. But those who were vaccinated developed eight to ten times the expected rate of a rare paralytic nervous system disorder, Guillain-Barre syndrome. Most of those stricken recovered within a few months, but several died, and the episode continues to haunt annual flu-vaccination campaigns. Public health officials dismiss the Guillain-Barre episode as a fluke. They say that since it occurred more than a decade ago, tens of millions of Americans have received flu vaccine without any serious side effects.

However, even if everyone were vaccinated, some people would still get the flu because the vaccine is only about 80 percent effective. Flu tends to be relatively mild in those who have been vaccinated.

Fortunately, type-A influenza can be successfully treated—and often prevented—with the prescription antiviral drug Symmetrel (amantadine hydrocholoride). Studies show that Symmetrel is 65 to 85 percent effective in preventing influenza A among the unvaccinated and that it hastens recovery if taken after the illness strikes. For people age ten to sixty-four (except those with kidney disease) the CDC recommends 100 milligrams of Symmetrel twice a day. Those over sixty-five should take 100 milligrams once a day. Consult your physician about dosages for children under ten. To prevent flu, Symmetrel must be taken every day during the local outbreak—usually for six to twelve weeks. To treat flu, start taking it as soon as possible after symptoms appear and continue taking it for forty-eight hours after symptoms disappear—usually for five to seven days. Compared with flu, Symmetrel causes only minor side effects. Five to 10 percent experience some insomnia, light-headedness, irritability, or difficulty concentrating. Symmetrel is effective *only* against influenza A and not against influenza B or any of the common-cold viruses. Orthodox physicians say that influenza unresponsive to Symmetrel should be treated like the common cold (see chapter 8).

Advocates of vitamin C for the common cold also endorse it for flu. Linus Pauling recommends 1,000 to 2,000 milligrams per day for prevention, and up to 10,000 milligrams per day for treatment. The only significant side effect is possible diarrhea (see chapter 9).

Folk remedies for flu parallel those discussed for the common cold in chapter 10: hot toddies and chicken soup. Liquids are especially important for any illness that causes fever, a hallmark of influenza A.

Herbalists treat influenza with many of the same botanicals they use to treat colds (see the herbs recommended for flu and its symptoms in chapter 11).

Traditional Chinese medicine makes no distinction between the common cold and flu and recommends treating both illnesses using acupressure points and herbal medicines (discussed in Chapter 12).

Homeopaths recommend some of the same medicines for colds and flu: Aconite, Belladonna, Ferrum phos., and Byronia. But for fever with weakness, headache, and chills up and down the back, they suggest Gelsemium, a microdose of yellow jasmine. They also recommend Oscillococcinum, a microdose of duck heart and liver, a leading OTC flu remedy in Europe. Oscillococcinum may be purchased at natural food stores or from the homeopathic pharmacies listed in the resources section of chapter 13.

Zinc has not been studied as a treatment for influenza. But since many cases are symptomatically indistinguishable from the common cold, its proponents recommend the mineral for any upper respiratory infection on the dose schedule discussed in chapter 14.

Interferon does not appear to be effective against flu, but scientists say that rimantadine, a chemical relative of Symmetrel, holds promise as a future treatment for influenza A.

The only flu symptom not discussed in previous chapters is diarrhea, rare in adults but fairly common in children. The major risk is dehydration. Treatment involves clear liquids (water, apple juice, 7-Up, and so on) to replace lost fluids, and the "BRAT" diet, an acronym for bananas, rice, applesauce, and toast. For severe diarrhea, use Kaopectate, available over-the-counter at pharmacies.

No matter how you deal with your upper respiratory infections, prevention is preferable to treatment. If you're at risk for flu complications or if you come into close daily contact with anyone in a high-risk group, get a flu shot every fall.

One final note: Technically, there is no such disease as "stomach flu." Although this term is widely used, influenza, the real flu, does not usually cause gastrointestinal symptoms, except for diarrhea in children. "Stomach flu" is usually viral gastroenteritis, which typically causes sudden fever, nausea, vomiting, and diarrhea, but not upper respiratory symptoms.

. . .

Strep Throat

Strep throat typically affects children age two to fourteen with peak incidence from age six to eight. It is caused by *Streptococcus* bacteria, small colonies of which inhabit about one-third of school-aged children's throats without causing infection. But when they do, symptoms include fever, abdominal pain, headache, and vomiting, then a sore throat severe enough to make swallowing difficult, and swollen lymph glands in the upper neck. The immune system sends white blood cells to fight the bacteria, and the debris from the battle appears as patches of whitish pus in the back of the throat and on the tonsils. A rough, pink-red rash may also appear, typically on the child's chest and abdomen. Years ago, the combination of this rash and the symptoms listed above was called scarlet fever. Then scientists learned that scarlet fever was simply a variant of strep infection.

Without treatment, the body usually heals itself within two weeks. However, in about one in two hundred to three hundred untreated cases, the child develops rheumatic fever, which may cause permanent heart damage, or a potentially serious kidney infection called glomerulonephritis. Because of the small but real risk of these complications, physicians take throat cultures when a child has strep symptoms, and if *Streptococcus* is identified, they prescribe either a ten-day course of penicillin, a single long-acting penicillin shot, or erythromycin for those allergic to penicillin.

Whooping Cough

Medically known as pertussis from the Latin for "intense cough," this childhood bacterial infection initially resembles the common cold, with fever, runny nose, sneezing, and cough. But the "cold" lingers, and after about two weeks, the child's nasal discharge thickens and the cough becomes more intense, with a "whoop" sound during inhalations after bursts of coughing.

If left untreated, whooping cough usually clears up within two weeks but may become very serious. Since it's caused by bacteria, antibiotics are usually effective but not always. In serious cases children are hospitalized to receive intravenous antibiotics. Fatalities are rare but possible.

Pneumonia is a fairly frequent complication of whooping cough, especially in infants and young children. Before whooping cough vaccine was developed, pertussis-related pneumonia was a frequent cause of infant and childhood death. Vaccination is recommended at two, four, six, and eighteen months, and at four years.

However, in recent years, the vaccine has come under fire because of its potential side effects. In an estimated one case in 100,000, it causes nervous system disorders, and in about one case in 300,000, it causes permanent neurological damage, usually involving mental retardation. Critics say whooping cough is no longer a threat in North America and that the vaccine's potential risks outweigh its benefits. As a result, many parents no longer have their children vaccinated, and whooping cough outbreaks have become somewhat more common in recent years.

Considerable bad press about pertussis vaccine's side effects in England led to a dramatic reduction in vaccinations there in the mid-1970s (a decline much more pronounced than the modest decline in the United States). A few years later, a whooping cough epidemic swept unvaccinated British infants and children, causing 100,000 cases of the disease and 20 deaths. Despite critics' misgivings, most physicians strongly support vaccination. (A new, safer pertussis vaccine is currently under development.)

. . .

Allergies

Allergies to pollen, dust, molds, animal dander, and other substances often cause itchy, watery eyes, runny nose, nasal congestion, and sneezing. Unlike cold symptoms, allergies recur seasonally and are closely associated with exposure to the offending substances—pets, gardens, and so forth. Symptoms are typically relieved by avoiding allergy triggers, taking antihistamines, or allergy shots.

Mumps

Mumps is a childhood viral disease that causes fever, headache, earache, and swollen salivary glands in the cheeks and under the jaw. The fever typically subsides within a week, the swollen glands within two. A vaccine administered at fifteen months confers lifelong immunity. Mumps is rarely serious in young children, but if an unvaccinated teenage boy or adult man catches it from contact with an infected child, the disease may spread to the testicles, causing severe pain and, in rare cases, infertility.

Meningitis

Meningitis is either a viral or a bacterial infection of the membranes that cover the brain and spinal cord. The bacterial form is the more serious; fortunately, it is treatable with antibiotics.

Bacterial meningitis strikes an estimated forty thousand children in the United States each year, with peak incidence from six to twelve months. Ninety percent of cases occur in children under five, but the disease may strike at any age.

Symptoms vary widely from the classic high fever, headache, and stiff neck, and often include typical upper respiratory complaints. As a result, diagnosis is difficult. In infants, suspicious signs include poor feeding, crying when cuddled, and crankiness when moved or held. In older children, in addition to fever and stiff neck, listlessness, confusion, and visual difficulties are common. Because death is possible, *anyone who develops fever and stiff neck should consult a physician immediately.*

Bacterial meningitis is diagnosed by examining a sample of cerebrospinal fluid obtained by inserting a needle into the spinal area (lumbar puncture). Unfortunately, previous treatment with antibiotics may confound the diagnosis by suppressing the bacterial count in this fluid. If bacterial meningitis is confirmed (or strongly suspected), it is treated with antibiotics.

The leading cause of bacterial meningitis is *Haemophilus influenzae* B (HIB—no relation to the influenza viruses). A recently developed vaccine is recommended at age two. The vaccine is 90 percent effective. It carries a 2 percent risk of local reaction, but no serious side effects have been reported.

Viral meningitis, often caused by an enterovirus (Coxsackie or echovirus), produces symptoms similar to bacterial meningitis, but no bacteria appear in the cerebrospinal fluid. Viral meningitis is usually mild, and the body heals itself within a few weeks. Treatment involves rest, acetaminophen, and fluids.

Fever and Rash in Children

Since many early-childhood diseases may cause fever, runny nose, and other cold symptoms, the early stages of a great many childhood illnesses may be mistaken for the common cold. Frequently, one distinguishing symptom is a rash, which usually appears within a day or two of the onset of the illness. Rash may signal measles, chicken pox, German measles (rubella), roseola, fifth disease, or scarlet fever (strep infection). Consult a physician for any fever/rash combination.

CHAPTER
19

My Favorite Cold Cures

No guide to the common cold would be complete without the author revealing his own approach to humanity's leading illness. I offer no "miracle cure," just a humble but heartfelt belief that a positive attitude and creative self-care can prevent many colds and substantially reduce the duration and severity of most of those that defy preventive efforts.

I started the research for this book in late 1984—not from any belief that I (or anybody) had The Answer to the common cold, but simply because the magazine I edit, *Medical Self-Care,* needed a consumer's guide to cold remedies for the 1984–85 cold and flu season. I felt fatalistic about the common cold. I believed the orthodox medical position that colds could neither be prevented nor cured and that symptomatic relief was the only alternative.

At the time, I suffered two to four colds a year, and my wife and I almost always passed our upper respiratory infections to each other. My self-care program, such as it was, involved:

- Cursing fate as the sore throat took hold.
- Denying the illness as much as possible.
- Dragging myself to work despite my misery.
- Taking generic single-action OTCs for my symptoms, which never seemed to do much.
- Cursing fate again for invariably turning my colds into lingering cases of bronchitis that dragged on, sometimes for weeks.

Colds depressed me. I felt angry at myself for getting sick and generally viewed upper respiratory infections as a sign of moral weakness. Oh sure, from time to time I tried other cold remedies—vitamin C, chicken soup, and various herb teas—but always in a desultory, disorganized fashion. Deep down, from the first twinge in my throat, I felt convinced that nothing on earth could spare me the misery I was about to endure.

Now I feel much differently.

For General Immune Enhancement

I don't smoke. In addition to the cancer and heart disease risk, smoking depletes the body of vitamin C, necessary for a healthy immune system, and increases the risk of cold complications.

Without being a dietary dogmatist, my diet generally follows the guidelines discussed in chapter 6: low fat and high fiber; light on red meats, fried foods, and rich desserts; heavy on whole grains, fresh fruits, and vegetables.

Some nutrition authorities say that this diet supplies enough of all necessary nutrients, but I'm one of the 70 million Americans who doesn't quite believe it. In addition to eating a healthy diet, I also take 1,000 milligrams of vitamin C daily and an "insurance formula" multivitamin and mineral supplement, which contains the other nutrients that enhance immune response: A, E, and the B vitamins.

My diet/supplementation program is an easy, low-cost way to maintain a healthy, ready-to-fight-colds immune system without enduring the expense or intricacies of the various so-called "immune boosting" diets and supplement regimens that have become popular in recent years. There's nothing wrong with many of these programs, but strip away the hype and they come down to minor variations on the diet I already follow.

To Prevent Transmission

As discussed in chapter 5, some cold researchers favor hand-to-hand transmission with self-inoculation while others endorse the aerosol route. The jury is still out, but it's a good bet that cold viruses maintain their position as humanity's number-one illness by spreading *both* ways—and possibly in ways that scientists have not even discovered.

Nonetheless, I've personally become a fan of the hand-to-hand, self-inoculation perspective. Don't get me wrong—I try my best to avoid everyone's cough and sneeze aerosols. But ever since my wife and I began avoiding hand-to-hand contact with cold sufferers; washing our hands frequently; using only paper tissues and separate bathroom cups, we have reduced the number of colds we pass back and forth. Granted, this is what scientists dismiss as "anecdotal evidence," but it seems to work for us.

At the First Sign of a Cold

Recall from chapters 3 and 4 that the body's first line of defense against the common cold is immunoglobulin A

(IgA) and that meditative relaxation exercises and "selfless love" boost IgA secretion and have significantly reduced cold susceptibility in well-designed studies.

In my opinion, cold prevention starts with a *positive attitude,* the conviction that "I don't have to get sick. Instead of giving in to this cold, I'm going to take action right now and beat it." The instant I feel any throat twinge, I no longer curse fate and resign myself to another damnable cold. Now I *immediately* stop what I'm doing and practice the relaxation/visualization exercises discussed in chapter 6. I meditate on my immune system's soon-to-be-victorious struggle against the cold. I visualize my neutrophils, macrophages, T-cells, B-cells, killer cells, interferons, interleukin-2, and complement proteins beating back the viral hordes.

While visualizing wholesale virucide, I promptly take several other steps to nip the cold in the bud. I find that cold prevention works best when practiced immediately with a coordinated, multifaceted approach.

• *I take zinc every two hours.* As George Eby recommends (see chapter 14), I suck on two 23-milligram zinc lozenges at the first sign of a sore throat, then one lozenge every two waking hours until my symptoms have cleared. The research in favor of zinc is scant, but I've been consistently impressed with the mineral. Many brands are available, but my favorite is Cold Season Plus (see resources). I also carry zinc with me when I travel.

• *I take 1,000 milligrams of vitamin C every two hours.* Vitamin C's ability to enhance immune functioning is well established. As a cold cure, it remains controversial, but ascorbic acid does no harm, and many well-designed studies show that it provides significant relief (see chapter 9). I reduce my dose if diarrhea develops.

• *Between self-medication with zinc and vitamin C, I drink a cup or two of herb tea every hour.* For incipient colds, almost any beverage blend will do. I'm a big believer in hot liquids. They soothe the throat and their heat just might impair some viral replication. I let the tea water boil for several minutes and inhale some of the steam, because increased relative humidity helps prevent colds (see chapter 4). While brewing and sipping my tea, I continue my visualizations.

• *I write a check to my favorite charity.* Financial generosity is not exactly the kind of selfless love shown to boost the immune system (see chapter 6), but it's close enough. After all, charity is its own reward, and if my T-cells draw strength from an act of not-quite-selfless love, so much the better.

• *I try to make a meal of chicken soup.* In addition to the research that shows chicken soup superior to hot water in speeding the clearance of nasal mucus (see chapter 10), being Jewish, I derive special comfort from my people's ethnic cold remedy.

• *In the evening, I drink hot toddies.* I never drink and drive, but once I'm home, I'm partial to a combination of an herb tea, lemon, honey, and well-aged cognac.

• *Finally, I go to bed early.*

During my years of common-cold fatalism, it was a rare sore throat that did not turn into a full-blown cold. Now about half to two-thirds of my proto-colds are gone by the next morning.

Treatment

Of course, despite my best preventive efforts, a few proto-colds still become true colds. When this happens, I continue the vitamin C, zinc, and chicken soup, but if I want symptomatic relief, I switch from a beverage-blend herb tea to one of the FDA-approved OTC blends produced by Traditional Medicinals (see resources). Savoring a medicinal herb tea feels more therapeutic than popping a pill. The steam increases the relative humidity, and the ritual of tea preparation creates time for more visualization of my immune system winning the Battle of the Nasopharynx. I find that my full-blown colds are milder than the ones I recall from my years of fatalism. They last only four or five days, instead of six to eight, and rarely turn into lingering bronchitis.

Find Your Own Cold Cures

My favorite cold cures are just that—*mine.* I make no claim that my self-care program is the only way to deal with the common cold, or even the best way. Although my regimen is based on the research in this book, I have conducted no double-blind trials, and no doubt many cold researchers and others with strong ideas about upper respiratory infections would take issue with some or all of my ideas. But as Rhett said to Scarlett, "Frankly, I don't give a damn." I *honestly believe* that this program works for me; therefore, as discussed in chapter 7, at a minimum it helps mobilize the self-healing placebo phenomenon, which by itself is about 30 percent effective.

Far be it from me to tell you how to treat your colds. I don't have all the answers. That's part of the self-care approach to healing. Self-care means familiarizing yourself with the available alternatives, then designing the program that makes the most sense to you.

There's a whole world of cold cures out there. Find the ones that work best for you. You *don't* have to catch that next cold. And if you can't prevent it, there's a great deal you can do to cure it.

RESOURCES

Cold Season Plus Zinc Lozenges. See resources, chapter 14.

Traditional Medicinals OTC Herb Teas. See "Resources," chapter 11.

APPENDIX

About Medical Self-Care *Magazine and the* Self-Care Catalog

Medical Self-Care is "the encyclopedia of self-health," according to the *Washington Post,* and "the *Consumer Reports* of health and wellness," according to the *Los Angeles Times.* The twelve-year-old award-winning bimonthly empowers readers to stay healthy and to save money on health services by becoming better informed, more assertive health consumers.

Drawing on the nation's top health experts and medical writers, *Medical Self-Care* provides authoritative information about both orthodox and alternative healing arts. Articles emphasize sound nutrition, women's health, disease prevention, stress management, pediatrics for parents, first aid, healthy aging, psychological well-being, fitness without injury, and how best to cope with common illnesses and chronic conditions. The magazine also publishes reviews of the best new self-care books and products.

Readers of *Cold Cures* may obtain a free sample copy by writing: *Medical Self-Care,* P.O. Box 1000, Point Reyes, Calif. 94956, or calling (415) 663-8462 during business hours Pacific time.

The *Self-Care Catalog* is filled with essential, but often hard-to-find, self-care products for health-active individuals and families. In addition to the products listed in the resources Sections throughout this book, the *Self-Care Catalog* offers the best back care products, relaxation tapes, first-aid kits, weight control items, home medical instruments, home fitness equipment, massage supplies, personal comfort enhancements, car seats and other baby products, and a variety of useful items for everything from insomnia and motion sickness to diabetes and asthma.

Readers of *Cold Cures* may obtain a free copy by writing *Self-Care Catalog,* 11 Chapel St., Augusta, Me. or calling (207) 622-5949 during business hours Pacific time.

Bibliography

Introduction

Couch, R. B. "The Common Cold: Control?" *Journal of Infectious Diseases* 150 (August 1984):167–73.

"Medical News." *Journal of the American Medical Association (JAMA)* 255 (January 17, 1986):301–306.

Roberts, C. R., et al. "Reducing Physician Visits for Colds Through Consumer Education." *JAMA* 250 (October 21, 1983):1986–89.

Chapter 1

Alexander, D. *The Common Cold and Common Sense.* New York: Fireside, 1971.

Murphy, W. *Coping with the Common Cold.* Alexandria, Va.: Time-Life Books, 1981.

Williams, R. L. "For the All-Too-Common Cold, We Are Perfect, If Unwilling, Hosts." *Smithsonian,* December 1983, pp. 47–55.

Chapter 2

Alexander, op. cit.

Murphy, op. cit.

Andrewes, C. H. "The Common Cold." *Scientific American* 184 (February 1951):39–45.

Dick, E. C., and S. C. Inhaorn. "Rhinoviruses." In *Textbook of Pediatric Infectious Diseases.* Edited by R. D. Feigin and J. D. Cherry. Philadelphia: W. B. Saunders, 1987, pp. 1539–1558.

Raeburn, P. "The Houdini Virus," *Science 85,* December 1985, pp. 52–57.

Horowitz, M. S., "Adenoviral Diseases," pp. 477–96; Melnick, J. L., "Enteroviruses, pp. 739–94; Couch, R. B. "Rhinoviruses," pp. 795–816; Chanock, R. M., and K. McIntosh, "Parainfluenza Viruses," pp. 1241–1254; McIntosh, K. and R. M. Chanock, "Respiratory Syncytial Virus," pp. 1285–1304; McIntosh, K. "Cornonaviruses," pp. 1323–31. In *Virology.* Edited by B. N. Fields. N.Y.: Raven Press, 1985.

Chapter 3

Murphy, op. cit.

Mizel, S. B., and P. Jaret. *The Human Immune System: The New Frontier in Medicine.* New York: Fireside, 1985.

Bellanti, J. A. *Immunology III.* Philadelphia: W. B. Saunders, 1985.

. . .

Chapter 4

Andrewes, op. cit.

Murphy, op. cit.

Dowling, H. F., et al. "Transmission of the Common Cold: The Effects of Chilling on Susceptibility." *American Journal of Hygiene* 68 (1958):59–65.

Muchmore, H. G., et al. "Persistent Parainfluenza Virus Shedding During Isolation at the South Pole." *Nature* 289 (January 15, 1981):187–89.

Berkman, S., and L. Syme. "Social Networks, Host Resistance, and Mortality." *American Journal of Epidemiology* 109 (1979):186–204.

Totman, R., et al. "Predicting Experimental Colds in Volunteers from Different Measures of Recent Life Stress." *Journal of Psychosomatic Research* 24 (1980):155–63.

Jacobs, M. A., et al. "Life Stress and Respiratory Illness," *Psychosomatic Medicine* 32 (May–June 1970):233–36.

Cluff, L. E., et al. "Asian Influenza: Infection, Disease, and Psychological Factors." *Archives of Internal Medicine* 117 (February 1966):159–63.

Chapter 5

Dochez, A. R., et al. "Experimental Transmission of the Common Cold by Means of a Filterable Agent." *Journal of Experimental Medicine* 52 (1930):701–16.

Wells, W. F., and W. R. Stone. "On Air-Borne Infection: Viability of Droplet Nuclei Infection." *American Journal of Hygiene* 20 (1934):619–27.

Andrewes, op. cit.

Dick and Chesney, op. cit.

Hendley, J. O., et al. "Transmission of Rhinovirus Colds by Self-Inoculation." *New England Journal of Medicine (NEJM)* 288 (June 28, 1973):1361–64.

Editorial, "Spread of Colds." *British Medical Journal,* October 20, 1973, pp. 123–24.

Editorial, "Where Do Cold Viruses Come From?" *The Lancet,* February 9, 1974, pp. 199–200.

Reed, S. E. "An Investigation of the Possible Transmission of Rhinovirus Colds Through Indirect Contact." *Cambridge Journal of Hygiene* 75 (1975):249–58.

D'Alessio, D. J., et al. "Transmission of Experimental Rhinovirus Colds in Volunteer Married Couples." *Journal of Infectious Diseases* 133 (January 1976):28–36.

Gwaltney, J. M., et al. "Hand-to-Hand Transmission of Rhinovirus Colds." *Annals of Internal Medicine* 88 (1978):463–67.

D'Alessio, D. J., et al. "Short-Duration Exposure and the Transmission of Rhinovirus Colds." *Journal of Infectious Diseases* 150 (August 1984):189–94.

Meschievitz, C. K., et al. "A Model for Obtaining Predictable Natural Transmission of Rhinoviruses in Human Volunteers." *Journal of Infectious Diseases* 150 (August 1984):195–201.

Dick, E. C., et al. "Interruption of Transmission of Rhinovirus Colds Among Human Volunteers Using Virucidal Paper Handkerchiefs." *Journal of Infectious Diseases* 153 (February 1986):352–56.

Dick, E. C., et al. "Aerosol Transmission of Rhinovirus Colds." *Journal of Infectious Diseases,* in press.

Fields, op. cit.

Chapter 6

Murphy, op. cit.

"Medical News." *JAMA* 255 (January 17, 1986):301–306.

Berger, Stuart M., M.D. *Dr. Berger's Immune Power Diet.* New York: Signet, 1985.

Dick, E. C., et al. "Lack of Increased Susceptibility to Colds in the McMurdo Winter Parties of 1975 and 1976." *Antarctic Journal of the U.S.* (1977), pp. 3–4.

Flynn, T. C., et al. "Colds and Immunity in the Winter Personnel at McMurdo, 1976." *Antarctic Journal of the U.S.* 12 (1977):5–6.

Dick, E. C., et al. "Possible Modification of the Normal Fly-In Respiratory Disease Outbreak at McMurdo Station." *Antarctic Journal of the U.S.* 15 (1980):173–74.

Dick, E. C., et al. "Interruption of Transmission of Rhinovirus Colds Among Human Volunteers Using Virucidal Paper Handkerchiefs." *Journal of Infectious Diseases* 153 (February 1986):352–56.

Hendley, J. O., et al. "Evaluation of Virucidal Compounds for Inactivation of Rhinovirus on Hands." *Antimicrobial Agents and Chemotherapy* 14 (November 1978):690–94.

Gwaltney, J. M., and J. O. Hendley. "Transmission of Experimental Rhinovirus Infection by Contaminated Surfaces." *American Journal of Epidemiology* 116 (1982):828–33.

Sobel, D. "The Positive Effects of Negative Ions." *Medical Self-Care,* Spring 1980, pp.:28–29.

Krueger, A. P., and E. J. Reed. "Biological Impact of Air Ions," *Science* 193 (September 24, 1976):1209–1213.

Green, R. G., et al. "Immunoenhancement: A Comparison of Four Relaxation Methods." *Psychosomatic Medicine* 48 (March–April 1986):304.

Borysenko, J. Z. "Healing Motives: An Interview with David C. McClelland." *Advances* 2 (Spring 1985):29–41.

Chapter 7

Beecher, H. K. "The Powerful Placebo." *JAMA* 159 (December 24, 1955):1602–1606.

Honigfeld, G. "Non-Specific Factors in Treatment: Review of Placebo Reactions and Placebo Reactors." *Diseases of the Nervous System* 25 (March 1964):145–56.

Honigfeld, G. "Non-Specific Factors in Treatment: Review of Social-Psychological Factors." *Diseases of the Nervous System* 25 (April 1964):225–39.

Levine, J. D., et al. "The Mechanism of Placebo Analgesia." *The Lancet,* September 23, 1978, pp. 654–57.

Evans, F. J. "Expectations and the Placebo Response." *Advances* 1 (Summer 1983):10–19.

Wickramasekera, I. "The Placebo as Conditioned Response." *Advances* 1 (Summer 1983):20–24.

Chapter 8

Zimmerman, D. R. *The Essential Guide to Nonprescription Drugs.* New York: Harper & Row, 1983.

Franklin, N. "Dubious Drugs for Coughs and Colds." *Medical Self-Care,* Summer 1982, pp. 38–41.

Graedon, J. and T. "Drugs and Alcohol Don't Mix." *Medical Self-Care,* November 1986, p. 17.

Stanley, E. D., et al. "Increased Virus Shedding with Aspirin Treatment of Rhinovirus Infection." *JAMA* 231 (March 24, 1975):1248–51.

West, S. W., et al. "A Review of Antihistamines and the Common Cold" *Pediatrics* 56 (July 1975):100–107.

Howard, J. C., et al. "Effectiveness of Antihistamines in the Symptomatic Management of the Common Cold." *JAMA* 242 (November 30, 1979):2414–17.

Napoli, M. "Cold and Flu Self-Care Guide." *Health Facts,* January 1985.

"Cold Self-Care Kit." Kaiser-Permanente, Vallejo, Calif., 1985.

Chapter 9

Pauling, L. *Vitamin C and the Common Cold and Flu.* San Francisco: W. H. Freeman, 1976.

Pauling, L. *How to Live Longer and Feel Better.* New York: W. H. Freeman, 1986.

"Ascorbic Acid and the Common Cold." *Nutrition Reviews* 25 (August 1967):228–31.

Anderson, T. W. "Vitamin C and the Common Cold: A Double-Blind Trial." *Canadian Medical Association Journal* 107 (September 23, 1972):503–508.

Hume, R., and E. Weyers. "Changes in Leucocyte Ascorbic Acid During the Common Cold." *Scottish Medical Journal* 18 (January 1973):3–7.

Coulehan, J. L., et al. "Vitamin C Prophylaxis in a Boarding School." *NEJM* 290 (January 13, 1974):6–10.

Anderson, T. W., et al. "Winter Illness and Vitamin C." *Canadian Medical Association Journal* 112 (April 5, 1975):823–26.

Campbell, G. D. "Ascorbic Acid-Induced Hemolysis in G-6-PD Deficiency." *Annals of Internal Medicine* 82 (June 1975):810.

Stein, H. D., et al. "Ascorbic Acid-Induced Uricosuria." *Annals of Internal Medicine* 84 (April 1976):385–88.

Coulehan, J. L., et al. "Vitamin C and Acute Illness in Navajo Schoolchildren." *NEJM* 295 (October 28, 1976):973–77.

Pinz, W., et al. "Effect of Ascorbic Acid Supplementation on the Human Immunological Defense System." *International Journal for Vitamin and Nutrition Research* 47 (1977):248–57.

Clemetson, C.A.B. "Histamine and Ascorbic Acid in Human Blood." *Journal of Nutrition* 110 (1980):662–68.

Anderson, R. "Ascorbate-Mediated Stimulation of Neutrophil Motility and Lymphocyte Transformation." *American Journal of Clinical Nutrition* 34 (September 1981):1906–1911.

Carr, A. B., et al. "Vitamin C and the Common Cold." *Medical Journal of Australia* 2 (October 17, 1981):411–12.

Kasa, R. M. "Vitamin C: From Scurvy to the Common Cold." *American Journal of Medical Technology* 49 (January 1983):23–26.

Ovesen, L. "Vitamin Therapy in the Absence of Obvious Deficiency." *Drugs* 27 (1984):148–70.

"Some Vitamin Myths." *Consumer Reports,* March 1986.

Malone, H. E., et al. "Ascorobic Acid Supplementation: Its Effects on Body Iron Stores and White Blood Cells." *Irish Journal of Medical Science* 155 (March 1986):74–79.

Chapter 10

Wilen, J. and L. *Chicken Soup and Other Folk Remedies.* New York: Fawcett Columbine, 1984.

Saketkhoo, K., et al. "Effects of Drinking Hot Water, Cold Water, and Chicken Soup on Nasal Mucus Velocity." *Chest* 74 (October 1978):408–410.

Chapter 11

Kaufman, R. M., and T. Siek. "Is 'Natural' Always Healthy?" *Journal of School Health,* August 1980, pp. 322–25.

Spoerke, D. G. "Herbal Medication: Use and Misuse." *Hospital Formulary,* December 1980, pp. 941–51.

McCaleb, R. S. "Herbal Safety." *Herb News,* Spring 1981, pp. 12–14.

Dittmar, M. J. "Herbal Renaissance." *Health Food Business,* April 1982, pp. 50–60.

"Herbs Hazardous to Your Health." *American Pharmacy* NS24 (March 1984):20–21.

"Survey: Herbs." *Natural Foods Merchandiser,* August 1984, pp. 54–57.

"Herbal Rx: Promoting Alternative OTC Drugs." *Natural Foods Merchandiser,* September 1984, pp. 18–25.

Sullivan, F. "Herbs: A Market Worth Cultivating." *Health Food Business,* August 1985, pp. 32–45.

Johnson, E. S., et al. "Efficacy of Feverfew as Prophylactic Treatment of Migraine." *British Medical Journal* 291 (August 31, 1985):569–72.

Duke, J. A. *CRC Handbook of Medicinal Herbs.* Boca Raton, Fla.: CRC Press, 1985.

Tierra, M. *The Way of Herbs.* New York: Washington Square Press, 1983.

Weiner, M. *Weiner's Herbal.* Briarcliff Manor, N.Y.: Stein & Day, 1980.

Spoerke, D. G. *Herbal Medications.* Santa Barbara, Calif.: Woodbridge Press, 1980.

Tyler, V. *The Honest Herbal.* Philadelphia: G. F. Stickley, 1983.

Chapter 12

Liu, H. "Treating Colds and Flu the Chinese Way, Part I." *Oklahoma State Medical Journal* 77 (September 1984):318–23.

Liu, H. "Treating Colds and Flu the Chinese Way, Part II." *Oklahoma State Medical Journal* 77 (October 1984):361–65.

Blate, M. *The Natural Healer's Acupressure Handbook.* Hollywood, Fla.: Falkynor Books, 1983.

Chang, S. T. *The Complete Book of Acupuncture.* Berkeley, Calif.: Celestial Arts, 1976.

Kaptchuk, T. *The Web That Has No Weaver: Understanding Chinese Medicine.* New York: Congdon & Weed, 1983.

Tierra, M. op. cit.

• • •

Chapter 13

Gibson, R. "Homeopathic Therapy in Rheumatoid Arthritis: A Double-Blind Clinical Trial." *British Journal of Clinical Pharmacology* 9 (1980):453–59.

Reilly, D. T. "Is Homeopathy a Placebo Response? A Controlled Trial in Hayfever." *The Lancet,* October 18, 1986, pp. 881–86.

Cummings, S., and D. Ullman. *Everybody's Guide to Homeopathic Medicines.* (Los Angeles: J. P. Tarcher, 1984).

Chapter 14

Eby, G., et al. "Reduction in Duration of Common Colds by Zinc Gluconate Lozenges in a Double-Blind Study." *Antimicrobial Agents and Chemotherapy* 25 (January 1984):20–24.

"Zinc and Colds." *Science News* 130 (October 11, 1986):238.

Samo, T. C., et al. "Intranasally Applied Recombinant Leukocyte A Interferon in Normal Volunteers: Minimal Effective and Tolerable Dose." *Journal of Infectious Diseases* 150 (August 1984):181–88.

Hayden, F. G., and J. M. Gwaltney. "Intranasal Interferon-A_2 Treatment of Experimental Rhinoviral Colds." *Journal of Infectious Diseases* 150 (August 1984):174–80.

Douglas, R. M., et al. "Prophylactic Efficacy of Intranasal A_2-Interferon Against Rhinovirus Infections in the Family Setting." *NEJM* 314 (January 9, 1986):65–70.

Hayden, F. G., et al. "Prevention of Natural Colds by Contact Prophylaxis with Intranasal A_2-Interferon." *NEJM* 314 (January 9, 1986):71–75.

Phillpotts, R.J. et al. "Activity of Enviroximine Against Rhinovirus Infection in Man." *The Lancet,* June 20, 1981, pp. 1342–1344.

Otto, M. J. et al. "In Vitro Activity of WIN 51711, A New Broad-Spectrum Antipicornavirus Drug." *Antimicrobial Agents and Chemotherapy,* 27 (June 1985):883–886.

Marwick, C. "Possible Defense Against Common Cold: 'Block That Cellular Receptor Site.'" *JAMA,* 256 (August 22, 1986):967–971.

Schmeck, H. M. "New Discovery Blocks Doorway For Cold Virus." *New York Times.* September 16, 1986 pp. 17–20.

Chapter 15

OTC Drug Committee. Coalition for the Medical Rights of Women. "Safe Natural Remedies for the Discomforts of Pregnancy." San Francisco: CMRW, 1982.

Sloane, P. D. et al. *The Complete Pregnancy Workbook.* Chapel Hill, N.C.: Algonquin Books, 1986.

Chapter 16

Spock, B. and M. B. Rothenberg. *Baby and Child Care.* New York: Pocket Books, 1985.

Pantell, R. H. et al. *Taking Care of Your Child.* Reading, Massachusetts: Addison-Wesley, 1984.

Samuels, M. and N. *The Well Child Book.* New York: Summit, 1982.

Clayman, C. B. and J. R. M. Kunz. *Children: How to Understand Their Symptoms.* New York: Random House, 1986.

"Reyes Syndrome, U.S., 1985." *JAMA,* 255 (March 21, 1986):1415–1416.

Chapter 17

Pantell, op. cit.

Samuels, op. cit.

Tapley, D. F. et al. *The Columbia University College of Physicians and Surgeons Complete Home Medical Guide.* New York: Crown, 1985.

Isselbacher, K. J. *Harrison's Principles of Internal Medicine,* 9th Ed. New York: McGraw Hill, 1980.

Chapter 18

Murphy, B. R. and R. G. Webster. "Influenza Viruses." pp. 1179–1240 in *Virology,* B. N. Fields et al, eds., New York: Raven Press, 1985.

Moser, M. R. et al. "An Outbreak of Influenza Aboard a Commercial Airliner." *American Journal of Epidemiology.* 110 (July 1979):1–6.

Perrotta, D. M. et al. "Acute Respiratory Disease Hospitalizations as a Measure of Epidemic Influenza." *American Journal of Epidemiology,* 122 (1985): 468–476.

"Update: Influenza and the Role of Rapid Virus Typing in Improving Amantadine Use, U.S." *JAMA,* 255 (February 14, 1986):728.

Centers for Disease Control, "Current Trends: Influenza, U.S." *Morbidity and Mortality Weekly Report,* 35 July 25, 1986:470–479.

Tapley, op. cit.

Isselbacher, op. cit.

Index

About the Author

Michael Castleman, M.A., editor of *Medical Self-Care* magazine, is an award-winning journalist, author, and screenwriter. His books include *Sexual Solutions* (1980) and *Crime Free* (1984), and *The Medical Self-Care Book of Women's Health* (1987, co-authored with Bobbie Hasselbring and Sadja Greenwood, M.D.). His films include the short subjects "Condom Sense" (1981) and "Hard Climb" (1983). He has also written for *The New York Times, Redbook, Self, Runner's World, The Nation, Sierra,* the *San Francisco Chronicle* and *Examiner,* and many other publications. He lives in San Francisco with his wife, Anne Simons, M.D., and son, Jeffrey.